FOREVER YOUNG

YOUR PERSONAL TRAINER

By

Frank and Karen Cuva

A Weight Training Guide for the Baby Boomers and Beyond

Forever Young Fitness Northridge, Ca. 91326
www.foreveryoung-fitness.com
email: cuvafitness@ sbcglobal.net

Copyright 2001
Library of Congress, Copyright Office
ISBN 0-9728221-0-0

Table of Contents

FORWARD

This book has come at the right time, with epidemics of obesity, rising incidence of diabetes, high blood pressure and dementia. At the same time, we have the largest increase of baby boomers reaching their senior years.

Everyone should stop and reassess their priorities.

It is essential to realize that the human body is not just a piece of biochemical machinery that deteriorates steadily over time. Rather, it is a magnificently organized and integrated interplay of spiritual, physical, chemical, informational and a psychological work of art. It is designed to last for at least one hundred fifty years. The key to realize the maximum potential of this equipment is with proper and timely maintenance by knowledgeable technicians to exploit each of these aspects to their maximum. This book is designed to assist you in one of these elements. The physical conditioning and maintenance of that marvelous machine--your body.

Who doesn't know the simple rule, *"Use it or lose it"*?

With new gadgets of entertainment like television, communication devices like cell phones, internet and beepers, coupled with means of commuting like cars, scooters and mopeds, we have eliminated even the meager use of our muscles. Associated with this, our technique of growing and distributing food has just about eliminated hunger, and our affluence has made it possible to easily afford the richest foods. On top of all this, we have advertisements showing us these sumptuous delicacies, tempting us to indulge ourselves to our hearts content. This deadly combination is the cause of this new epidemic, obesity.

We need to attack this enemy effectively. The idea of taking charge of your own health has gained acceptance, and claims about how to achieve wellness have proliferated.

Television and print media bombard us with information about gadgets for exercise. Their models with exquisite bodies make the entire workout appears so easy and they promise the desired results in six weeks. What hog wash! These models have used the techniques shown in this book for several years to create and maintain their physique. It is a lie. There is no quick fix, "No pain...No gain!"

Although awareness is the essential first step in any transformation, execution of knowledge is the only way to reap the actual benefit.

By applying the carefully chosen methods presented in these pages, you will experience a profound change in the quality of your lives, and avoid disabling injuries to achieve it. You will notice an immediate change in your physical and emotional well-being and reclaim the ability to tap into your inner reservoir of energy, vitality, and happiness. The physical change will take time, and it will happen, but so slowly that you might not even notice it. Others will see it before you do. So don't give up after a week or a month, work at it for six months. The change you appreciate will be your next driving force to continue. These six months of training, and the life style change they create, will buy you happiness for the rest of your life.

Misconceptions about weight lifting are:

• *"If a woman trains with weights, she will appear to be masculine or look like a professional body builder."* Chances of that happening are very remote. Women naturally carry more body fat than men. That is because it takes a certain amount of body fat for child bearing. That fat is what gives them that soft feminine look. That "body builder hard look" comes with extreme dieting and very rigorous hard work.

• *"I am too old to lift weights"* myth is common and needs to be addressed. Let me try to explain. Weight lifting is the best way to build muscles. That in turn, not only helps your strength but also increases the Basal Metabolic Rate, in short BMR. BMR is the measure of calories our body uses while our body is at rest (watching TV or sleeping). For every one pound of muscle growth, you increase your BMR fifty calories a day. This is equivalent to fifteen minutes of walking. So if you added only four pounds of muscle to your body, you have given yourself the benefit of walking one hour a day without actual walking. Isn't this perfect for a busy executive or a couch potato?

"Forever Young Your Personal Trainer" is designed as manual of renewal. A comprehensive resource that focuses on methods. In these pages you will find a simple and practical step-by-step program for reversing aging and resetting your biostat. You can implement this program right away. There are no gimmicks. It contains proven methods that have years of experience behind them.

The format of the book is user-friendly, with a ring binder, well illustrated with photos, and detailed text for easy understanding. The technique has been tested for all ages, particularly for the baby boomers. This should not stay on the shelf, but in your gym, den, or wherever you exercise.

Helping people to bring about this change has always been the goal of the Cuvas. To that end this book was conceived. Their intention was to create a publication that would clarify conflicting and superficial information presented by popular media. One of the crucial tenets is, preventing an ailment is just as important as curing it...perhaps more important. As a physician I can assure you that regular use of these exercises will delay or prevent osteoporosis, hip fractures, diabetes and dementia. It will improve sexual performance, memory, balance, and sleep. In the pages to follow you will find the nectar of youth.

Let us look at later part of our life as an opportunity for greater wisdom, creativity, meaning, love, emotional stability and physical fitness. The Cuvas have given you a blue print with this manual to live into the nineties, hundreds and beyond with sound bodies and clearer minds.

You can influence your health and well being through the choices you make. This book will prove to be a timeless classic in the field of physical exercise in times to come.

By,

Kant Tucker, MD

- Chairman and President of Kidney Centers, Inc.
- Former member of the Scientific Advisory Council of the National Kidney Foundation, Southern California Chapter.

Proper Nutrition
Aerobics
Weights

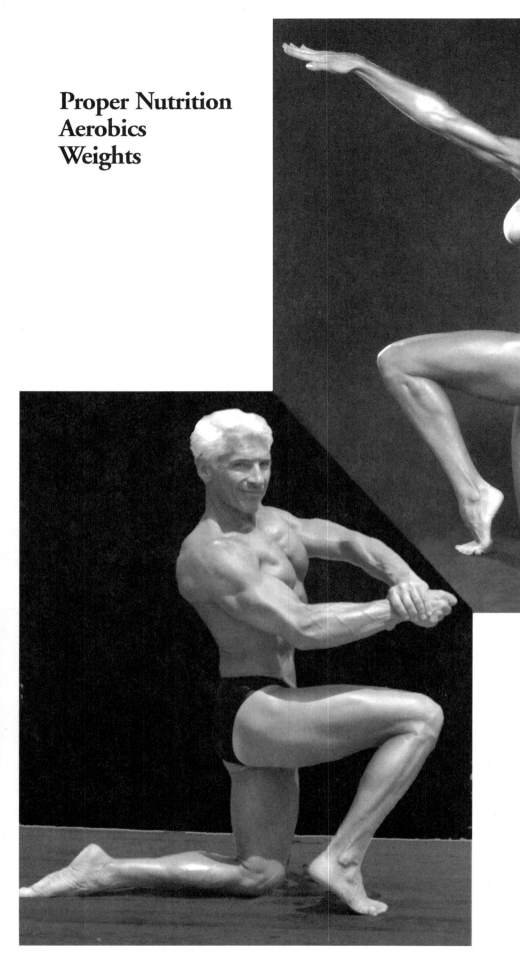

Achievable Goals
Determination
Consistancy

CHAPTER 1

WHY ANOTHER FITNESS MANUAL?

Recently, I was listening to a radio report that stated when a survey was taken of some thousands of adults, the question was asked, "If you could live to be a hundred and fifty years of age, would you want to?" I'm sure you figured out that most people said no. If you're over fifty and have touches of arthritis, lower back pain, skin problems, foot irritations or any of the hundreds of things that plague us as we grow older, you would have to agree with those that chose the negative.

However, if that surveyor had asked, "If you could live to be a hundred fifty years and were as productive and energetic as you were at forty," I feel quite certain your answer would have been, "you betcha I would!"

From all medical indications of the news media lately, the chance of living that one hundred fifty years is not that far off. It doesn't take a rocket scientist to figure out if you are one of the baby boomers, (which means you are about fifty at the time of this writing) you will live to be close to one hundred years of age. If you look around at the hundred year old people you have seen or met, that thought can't be very appealing to you.

It doesn't have to be that way, and that's why this manual was written. You know the answer to beating old age. Everyone does. Exercise and proper nutrition can, (and have), held back the ravages of time. Nutritional facts have been pounded into everyone's head from all sources of news media. Forget the ridiculous promises of people selling you a fast fix. In this book we will go over some simple facts about nutrition, but nothing you can't get for free from the government. Exercise manuals, magazines and tapes appear at every shopping mall, grocery store and health food store across the continent but few address the population over fifty and fewer still without a host of products they are trying to sell you for that "quick fix" that will instantly make you healthier and more beautiful in just a few short weeks.

There is no quick fix. The body wasn't built that way. It takes time and commitment to change the way you look and feel. If you are willing to make that kind of commitment, it is amazing how much you really can improve your body.

To start off let's make some realistic evaluations. We are not all created equal. Many of us look at Arnold Schwarzenegger or Cory Everson and think, "if I just train regularly and intensely, I can wind up looking like that". Unless you are a "genetic superior", that's a pretty unrealistic goal. A "genetic superior" is a person that is so gifted physically that any exercise they do, and food they eat is converted to muscle. Most of us do not fit into that category. Certainly my wife, Karen, and I don't fit into that slot.

That is not to say these "super-bodies" do not have to work to get the bodies they have. They do put long hard hours in the gym to acquire the muscle mass they attain. The point is the average person can train just as hard, put as much time in the gym and will in no way approach the gigantic size these "super-genetics" display. We can, however, improve the body we were born with and even more importantly, we can use those extra years of life productively for our efforts.

One thing I know for sure. We cannot improve by following the advice offered in the high powered ads. I was fortunate enough to see two very good examples of how true the ads were that we continually see in the fitness magazines.

The first case was a very famous physique star shortly after he won a National Title that qualified him to compete as a professional body builder. At a seminar I attended in Detroit, Michigan, he was asked how much protein powder he took to get in shape for the Nationals. His answer, "In all honesty I never took any supplements until they paid me to endorse them."

There is a lovely lady on ESPN that demonstrates how to exercise with weights. She was hired strictly from seeing her photographs. She had to know how to demonstrate the exercises so she came to our Studio to find out how to train with resistant type equipment. She had never used weights before coming to our gym!

While training here she asked us if we had ever tasted a certain "perfect food" supplement that was the current rage of all the Hollywood crowd. We said we had, and found it useless for us. When we inquired why she asked, she replied "Well I've just been hired to be on their team and I've never tasted the stuff!"

The only reason I mention this is that I have seen so many people beat themselves up because they fall short of goals that were impossible to reach in the first place. The body is a marvelous piece of work, but it does have it's limits. No matter how hard we try we can just do so much.

Years ago I trained show horses for a living. I rode almost all seats. That means I rode English, Western, Driving, Dressage, and some Jumping, but my favorite riding seat was Dressage.

At the time, my personal horse was an Appaloosa gelding named Dancer. He was a big horse, over sixteen hands tall and about fourteen hundred pounds. His coloring was white with black spots so he had the coloring of a typical Dalmatian dog. I tried my best to make him a winning Dressage horse. We worked long hard hours to give him that magical, elegant look that only these ballet dancers of the horse world possess.

Unfortunately, Dancer was meant to be a pleasure horse. He would work his heart out to please me and do whatever I asked. This beautiful animal was obedient and supple, but he was not a Dressage horse. The result of all our efforts was pulled muscles and long periods of lameness for him until I finally let him be what he was meant to be, a magnificent pleasure horse in the show ring and a joy to ride on the trail. This manual was designed to reach that potential you were born with.

The observations and suggestions in this Manual were developed over the last fifteen years in which we have been personal trainers. In our club, FOREVER YOUNG

FITNESS STUDIO, we have put in thousands of hours training people of all ages and backgrounds. With our experiences training clients from preteens to octogenarians, from housewives to CEO's of large corporations, we have gained a wealth of knowledge and training experience.

Some of these observations have been in stark contrast to statements from research centers. For example, one university program headed by a former "star" athlete stated people in their seventies and eighties could increase their strength and muscle mass by doing three sets of exercises per body part doing ten repetitions with heavy weights. In theory it might work, but in practical application we find that program of repetitive sets of the same exercise for the same body part wind up injuring the practitioner. Back injuries, elbow problems, hip pain and rotator cuff impingements, are some of the problems these older trainees experienced using this type of workout. Not only did they not make any physical gains, they became discouraged and gave up on the training!

On the other hand, we have found that a circuit training program was far more productive, very little chance of injury, much easier on the nervous system, and our clients enjoyed the workout!

A circuit training workout is one in which you go from one muscle group to a different muscle group with very little rest between sets. For example, you might do a chest exercise followed by a back movement followed by a calf exercise. This way a muscle is not worked so hard that it doesn't have a chance to recover. We have excellent results with people over sixty with this type of routine as well as with the younger people who want to lose weight or just simply desire to toughen up for the more arduous workouts.

Another observation we have noticed here in our studio is, if you want to use exercise to make the hundred year mark in good shape, the workouts must be fun. If you force yourself into the gym because you think this is something you have to do...forget it! You will give up in a very short time. It's true there is the break-in time which a person may or may not enjoy the workouts. However, if you are training properly and have the right attitude, in a few short weeks you will be looking forward to your sessions at the gym.

I've been working out since I was twelve years old, and I'm sixty-five at the time of this writing. I still look forward to my sessions with the weights and while I've changed my method of training because of the aging factor, hopefully, I will be battling the barbells for another thirty-five years!

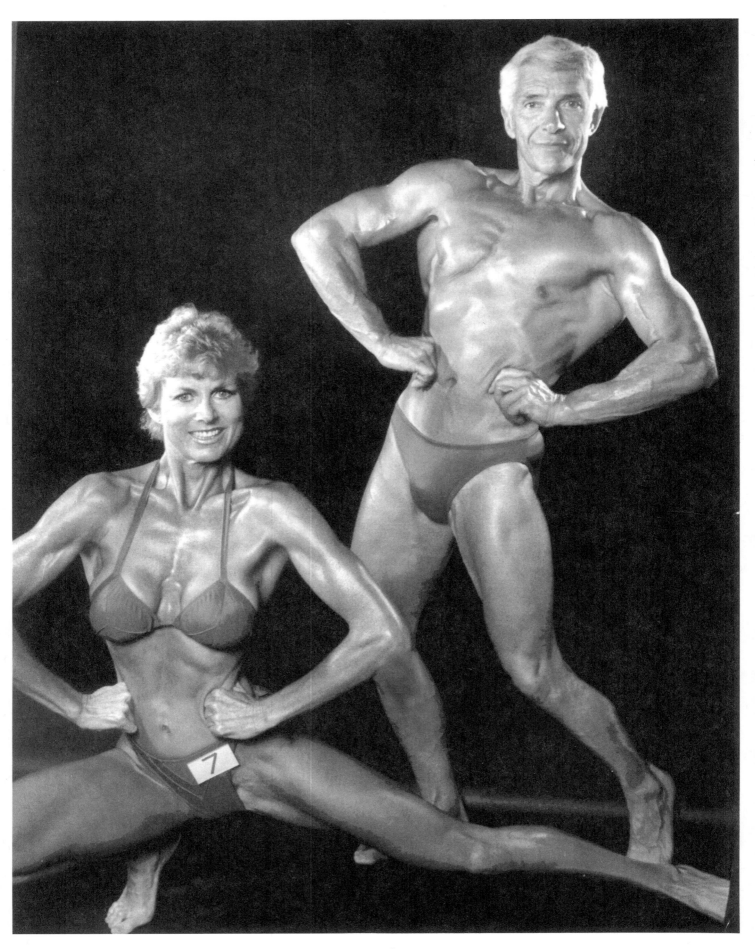

CHAPTER TWO

WHO WE ARE

It's difficult to believe I started training with weights over half a century ago! I can still remember as a child seeing the "Charles Atlas" ads in all the magazines and comics showing this dynamic muscular figure. He ran ads about this ninety-seven-pound weakling who was always getting sand kicked in his face when he was at the beach. Atlas claimed if you used his system of training no one would ever kick sand in your face again. I don't ever remember being a mere ninety-seven pounds but as a child I had lots of sand kicked at my face.

At twelve years of age I was about one hundred and sixty pounds and had a waist larger than my chest. I grew up in a neighborhood that consisted mainly of Italians and Afro-Americans. It was a tough area, and I had the misfortune of being part of a family that always tried to dress well and be socially correct. In grammar school I was subjected to beatings by my less conscientious fellow students who were more street wise than I was.

There was a problem at home as well. Like the celebrated actor and martial arts expert Chuck Norris, (and so many more children in these times), I had an abusive father with a drinking problem. When he drank too much, (and sometimes not too much) he got mean and started beating on the family. His target was always my mother, but my brother, sisters and I got our share of his displeasure as well.

One day at a drugstore magazine rack I saw this incredible muscular man on the cover of a magazine called "Strength and Health" and my whole life changed. I wanted to start lifting weights immediately, and despite my parents discouraging comments and refusing to purchase any equipment for me I decided to become a weight lifter. Dumbbells and barbells could be made from tin cans and cement. So armed with my homemade weights and an issue a month of "Strength and Health" magazine, I started my quest for that Herculean body.

A year after I started training, I had a confrontation with one of the bullies that had used me for a punching bag for a few years. I was outside in my backyard working out with my homemade weights, and he started picking on me. When he took a swing at me, I picked him up and threw him into the garage door. After he crawled up from the ground, he looked at me for a moment than walked away and never confronted me again.

Though I am not belligerent by nature, I did have some battles in the remainder of my school years but usually one blow was enough to discourage anyone from continuing to fight me. When I was sixteen, I was bench pressing over three hundred pounds and squatting with three hundred and fifty pounds.

At seventeen, I had my final confrontation with my father. He was drunk and in a mean mood. He started for my mother, and I stepped between them. I calmly said, "no more hitting." He looked at me for a moment then turned away, and he

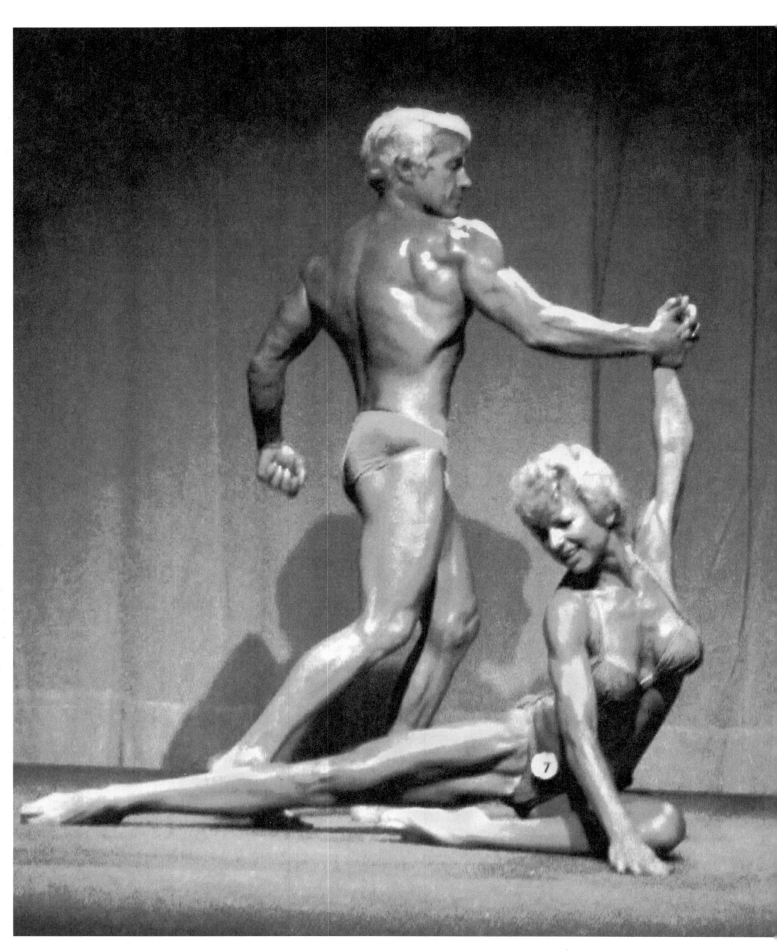

never struck any of us again. If I never won a physique contest or broke any lifting records, that moment made all the years of training worth the effort. Like the old Charles Atlas adds boasted, the "Sand Kicking" days were over.

There were lots of other challenges after that. The discipline I developed training so regularly, and dieting so conscientiously helped me overcome most of the obstacles I ran into and made it possible for me to enjoy the good times even more.

I trained regularly until I was about thirty-two. Then I became involved with other activities one of which was training horses. Horses became all consuming and I became so good at it that people paid me to train their horses, and before I knew it, sixteen years had slipped by.

Most people would think handling horses all day, building barns and shelters, laying pipes for drinking faucets, and shoveling tons of horse manure, would have kept my body in great shape. No such luck! The body adapts to any activity done on a regular basis. In fact, my body deteriorated so badly, I was having crippling back spasms a couple of times a year. My hands had developed arthritis so bad, I was constantly rubbing them to relieve the pain.

Nothing seemed to help until I decided to start training with the weights again. At first, the going was really rough. I was so weak I had to use weights that once were toys for me! As a youth I regularly used three hundred pounds in the bench press. Starting over again as a middle aged man of forty-eight, I could barely get ten repetitions with one hundred pounds. I was shocked that I had become so weak!

The discipline I had developed as a youth kept me coming back to the gym. Slowly the magic of the gym fired me up again. I loved watching the big muscle guys working out, bringing back fond memories of my youth. The banging of the heavy weights was music to my ears.

To my surprise and joy in a month's time my hands were back to normal. The pain was all gone! The back responded as well. I have not experienced a crippling back spasm since I returned to working out with the weights. Within two years I was back in physique competition in the Master's class.

Karen's story is quite different from mine. Though she too had the fat genes, her biggest problem was her extreme shyness. She has told me she was so shy when teachers called on her to give a report or answer a question in class, she would never stand up to recite her answers. She was too self-conscious to stand up in front of a group of people.

When we first started seeing each other Karen was eighteen years old. Back then, I must have done most of the talking. When we'd go to her company parties, if she said two sentences for the evening it was a big night for her. She was so pretty and sweet it didn't bother me.

The years slipped by and before we knew it she was thirty-three and struggling to get into a size fourteen pair of jeans. One night while we were watching home

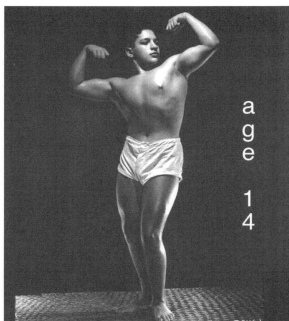

age 14

age 18

Through the Years

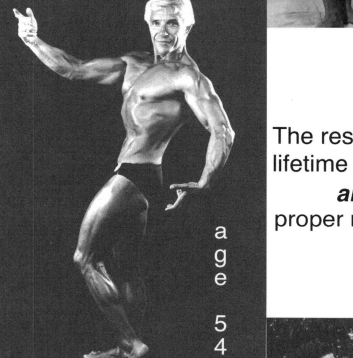

age 54

The results of a
lifetime of exercise
and
proper nutrition

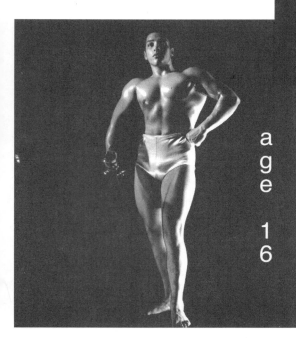

age 16

age 20

movies with my mother a picture of Karen walking away from the camera flashed across the screen, and my mother exclaimed, "I know who that is by the size of her butt."

That did it! She resolved to lose weight and get back into her youthful figure again. She was sure aerobics was the answer to her problem. Karen was born under the sign of Sagittarius. So with typical Sagittarian determination, she aimed her bow and let loose the arrow that changed her life.

In our living room for a full year she jumped and twisted and stretched according to the best information she could find. She got so good at it she gained enough confidence to go on Jack LaLanne's T.V. Show, and do his aerobics class live before the cameras. Part of Jack's program was to go through the group making individual comments on the participants, when he came to Karen he said, "This one is a twelve! That's two better than a perfect ten." The year of exercise was beginning to pay off!

While her progress had been good with the aerobic workouts, she was just a smaller version of what she was before she started exercising. Karen noticed I not only lost weight, but my whole appearance had changed. My shoulders and chest were larger and tighter while my waist was smaller and harder. So we hit the weights together. With the resistant type of workout, her body improved so fast that within a few months of pushing the weights, people in the gym were encouraging her to go into bodybuilding competition. I couldn't help thinking, "Karen, on a stage in front of a crowd of people in a bikini...impossible!"

As she continued to improve, competition became more and more appealing to both Karen and me. I had already brought home a couple of trophies from the Masters' classes and had a chance to observe the female contestants. Competition for women was still a new thing in the body building field. No one really knew what to look for in a female competitor.

Contests are not easy. It means hours of intense training and preparation. I knew once Karen made up her mind, she would stick to all training principles with dedication and tenacity. I encouraged her to go for it. Though the thought of getting out there on a stage all by herself was intimidating, she made the decision to take the plunge. Time was allotted for weight lifting, aerobics, posing and tanning. Motivation can work wonders. Of course, she still had to work at her job as well as do her everyday chores. For the next few years of competition, she averaged five hours nightly for sleep.

At her first contest, a local show in the San Fernando Valley, she came in third place and got her first trophy. The Daily News covered the event and used Karen's photo from the contest in their Life section. They also included a story on her views and training ideas for this new life-style.

With a placing to her credit, Karen decided to get real serious. Everyone at the gym was talking body fat so we sought out a place that did body composition test-

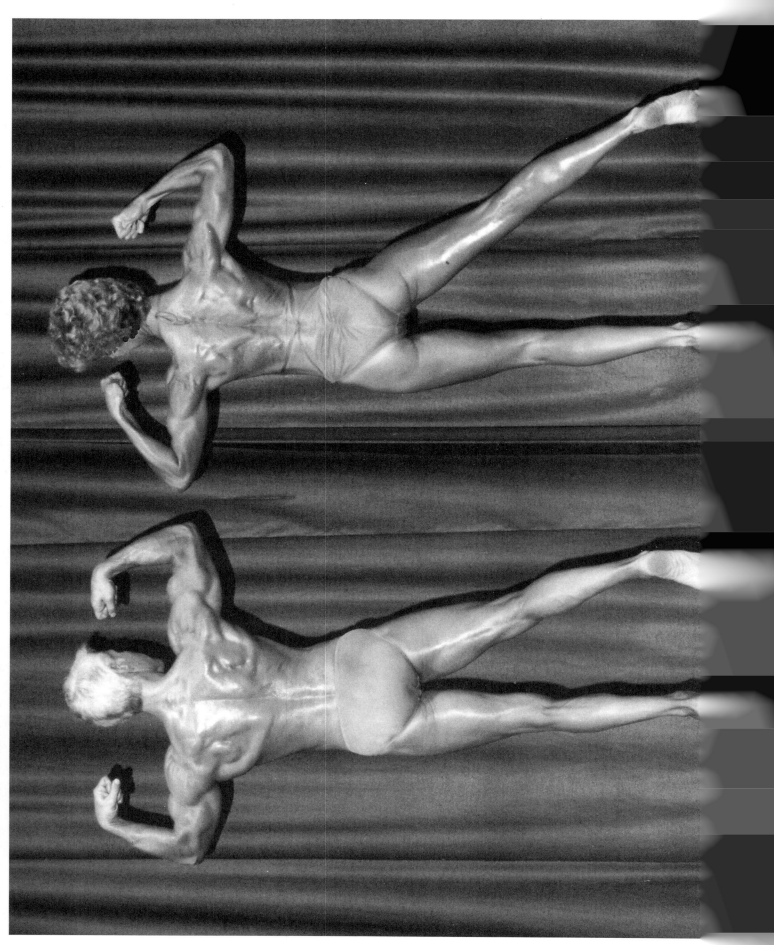

ing. The way to be defined enough to be competitive was to cut the body fat way down. We believed we were in excellent condition from all the training. The people administering the test thought we had to be pretty lean...but lo and behold we were still fat!

Unfortunately, we did not keep those original test scores. The method used was Hydrostatic weighing. That is, you are dunked in a tank of water three times then your score is averaged and they give you the results. I came in at fourteen percent and Karen came in at twenty-two percent body fat. Those were normal readings for a healthy person in that age bracket but hardly impressive for body-building competition.

The result of the test was to send us back to the drawing board, and it forced us to look into nutrition. Fat was out; protein was in with the vegetables and grains as our prime source of carbohydrates and fats. Our goals were ten grams of fat per day and one gram of protein per pound of body weight with lean carbohydrates completing the balance of allowed calories.

The plan worked! With combination of aerobic work, strict nutritional practices and the weights six days a week we both dropped into the athletes range. Karen competed in seventeen competitions that year, winning most of them. Between the two of us we won over fifty trophies in the next three years!

The big show on this part of sunny California was the Golden Valley Physique Classic. This competition always had a big turnout of quality contestants and that year was one of the biggest turnouts they had ever had up to that time. Karen walked away with top honors winning her height class and then the overall trophy.

That year the Amateur Athletic Union's Ms. America competition was held in Pasadena California and Karen had qualified to compete. After a really intense program and cutting her body fat as low as it has ever been, she wound up in the top three in the competition. The lady that won was more muscular than Karen, but I'm sure many felt Karen was definitely the most femininely fit woman in the competition.

Our final competition was in 1990 in Nobeoka, Japan where we had been invited to compete in the International Natural Body Building Championships. All of our competitions have been against drug free competitors. At that contest we were the oldest couple in the show. Karen was forty-three, and I was fifty-eight. Though she was almost twice as old as the nearest competitor, she finished third in this international show. I only garnered an honorable mention, but we had a great time, and we loved Japan.

Couples competition was our favorite event. We beat some great couples. Talk about togetherness! We posed to the sounds of "Memories" from the musical "Cats". I still can feel our moving together on the stage whenever I hear those haunting refrains. First place trophies are nice, but they are really just confirmation that the time and effort you put into your training was right and productive.

The reason for going over the stories of our competitive days was not to impress you with our showings but rather to bring out the incredible change that exercise made in our everyday lives. Karen went from a child afraid to stand up in school to recite her class assignments to a woman who has appeared on T.V. giving advice on training with weights, and lecturing in auditoriums, and competing in body-building on an international level. What she loves most, though, is the one on one personal training we have been doing over the years.

I went from a fat little boy, inept at any athletic endeavor, (who was used regularly for a punching bag), to a man that broke all the battalion physical fitness test records when I was drafted into the Korean Conflict. I have had many tests of strength and courage during my lifetime. Three times in my life I have had to do battle with leaders of youthful gangs and three times the gangs backed down.

For many years I trained Show horses. My specialty was training 'trouble horses". A "trouble horse" is an animal with bad habits that frighten its owner. You can imagine the strength and skill it takes to make a twelve hundred pound horse do something he doesn't want to do.

I detailed the metamorphosis Karen and I went through, to illustrate to you what two people who did not have a great beginning can do if they have the motivation and determination to CHANGE their lives.

There was nothing magical about what we accomplished. All it takes is a willingness to improve the condition of your body and the discipline to follow a common sense program to achieve that goal. This Manual was written to give you that plan.

CHAPTER THREE

HOW THE MUSCLES WORK

The body is a marvelous machine. Not only is it beautiful to behold when it is properly maintained, but it is extremely adaptable to almost any condition it runs into, and it is always trying it's best to be energy efficient.

The contours of the body are determined by the conditions of the muscles. Usually, the more muscular the body the more attractive it is to the general public. More importantly, the physically fit person can better perform the everyday tasks we all run into.

Each muscle consists of a multitude of fibers. The body is so efficient at conserving energy, only those fibers necessary to complete a movement will be utilized to execute that move. Not one fiber more, not one fiber less will be called upon to exercise an action.

Nature designed the body so that only the fittest will survive and be able to reproduce themselves. Unlike other animals, man could reason: and because of this unique ability, he was able to change things around enough so that it was not necessary to be a first class hunter to be able to survive. Physically though, the old principal still applies. So if you want to remain efficient, want to stave off predators, want to enjoy life despite the aging process, you must stay fit.

The good news is muscles never stop responding to exercise. If you are ninety and still exercise, the muscles will respond to your efforts. The bad news is the ligaments, and tendons are not so forgiving. They do become brittle with time so any workout has to take this into consideration as we grow older.

In order for muscles to grow they must be stressed. If no demands are made on a muscle, it will simply perform the movement as a natural part of it's everyday existence. However, if you make demands on the body that it is not accustomed to, it has to adjust so that if this task repeats itself, the body will be able to handle the movement easier the second time.

When a muscle is used, the fibers of those muscles extend and contract. The body is so efficient that only those fibers necessary to execute that movement will be involved. "Not one fiber more, not one fiber less will be utilized". When the muscle is stressed the fibers thicken as they contract. It is the thickening of these fibers that cause muscles to get stronger and larger. This process of the fibers thickening and causing them to grow so that they can handle the stress placed upon them is called <u>hypertrophy</u>.

So often a person will come into the studio and tell us they have been on a program where they are doing three sets of ten repetitions per set with the same weight. They may do several different exercises for a specific body part, but always with the three sets, ten reps program. When asked how much did you increase the weight since you started your program, invariably the answer is, "Well, I'm still using the same amount."

There cannot be any progress on such a program because there must be stress for the muscles to respond. As the exercise guru Jack LaLane states, "You must constantly challenge the body for it to get stronger." If you can handle the same weight for the same number of sets and the same number of repetitions every time, where is the stress? Remember, without any straining there is no thickening of the muscle fibers. Without hypertrophy you will not see any gains.

Stressing the muscle simply means you must go to failure at the completion of the movement. Failure means you cannot do another repetition in good form no matter how hard you try. If you went to failure on the first set, you would have to take a long rest to repeat the weight and count on the second set. If you went to failure on the second set, even after a very long rest, I doubt you could repeat the feat a third time.

It would be more productive to do one set with a weight that can be handled easily on the first set to warm up the muscle group. The second set should be difficult to get out the ten repetitions, but you do it. The third set should be a weight so heavy you could only do ten reps with the help of a training partner, and even then you should have difficulty getting eight repetitions. Under this scenario the muscle is truly taxed, and if followed rigorously will produce muscle size and strength.

Here at Forever Young Fitness Studio people are often surprised we change the training routines about every four weeks. Amazingly, people come to our studio that have been training for six, sometimes seven years without any change in their program. I have yet to see anyone on such a program that looked like an athlete.

The body is extremely adaptable. After a few weeks it is already adapting to the strain place upon it by an exercise. If doing hard repetitive movements produced an outstanding physique, every person who had a hard physical job would be muscular. Ever take a look at the guys holding those jack hammers breaking up the streets? How about gardeners digging ditches to lay pipe for a watering system? Not exactly Arnold Schwarzenegger. The first month on the job their bodies had already adapted to the work.

For muscles to grow, the work must be progressively more difficult. Just increasing the resistance is not enough. Different fibers and connecting tissues within the muscle react to changes in the positioning of the weight, the speed that a movement is executed, the rest between exercises, the type of equipment, and even the repetitions within a set. The more variety in the workout plan, the faster the results.

A great many competitive bodybuilders today change their workouts every two weeks. Many do split routines that work different body parts during the week.

In this way they can work a muscle group with more intensity in the training session and allow themselves more time for the muscle to recover. A muscle must have time to recover if it is to gain size and strength.

Growth does not take place while you are working out. In fact, muscles grow when you are resting. A serious bodybuilder must allow time so that the body can recover from the strain it has gone through during the workout. As we grow older, more time must be allowed for the body to recover. Three times a week at the gym for an hour is as much as most people can take if they are working out with sufficient intensity.

Friends that tell you they are working out for three hours five times a week, are socializing for most of that time...or they are on drugs. Taking steroids will allow a person to work out harder with less recovery time. That's great...if you are willing to take the heart, liver, and skin problems that go along with the use of steroidal type drugs. I have run into few people who can work out hard for more than an hour. Fewer still that can exercise for an hour and a half.

The primary source of energy for a workout comes from glycogen. Glycogen is manufactured in the body from carbohydrates. We all have a very limited supply of this substance. If you are extremely tired after a workout, you are experiencing a sugar low. This condition is caused by a complete depletion of the glycogen in your body. A carbohydrate meal after your workout will return you to a normal condition.

For increased growth and strength the muscles must be stressed. Muscles need time to recover. A sufficient amount of rest must be allowed between workouts. Most people will find working out three times a week for about an hour at a time will be sufficient for their bodies to respond properly to a progressive resistance exercise program with weights. Changing the program regularly will keep the body alert and ready to increase your strength for unexpected demands. The frequent changes will also keep the work interesting and make the work challenging and fun!

CHAPTER FOUR

THAT HORRIBLE WORD---DIET!

All diets work! At least for me they do. I have tried the high fat low carb diet. I have tried the egg and grapefruit diet, the one meal a day plan, the all rice diet, the high carb and low fat diet, the diet drink plan, and on and on, over the fifty years I have been involved with physical fitness.

The reason they all worked is because once I found the body weight I was pleased with, I never allowed myself to get more than five pounds above that weight. It must work. I have been within five pounds of my desired weight for over forty years. Getting to that desired weight is the trick!

Oprah Winfrey had a show once where she interviewed a group of people who had lost over one-hundred pounds of body weight and kept it off for over a year. They all had a couple of things in common. Everyone of them had tried a special fast weight lost program. Every one of them had gone through the YO-YO thing where they lose the weight and then gain it back plus a few pounds more. The most important thing this group had in common was they all agreed that once they made up their mind to really lose the weight it was not that hard to do.

None of this group had gone on any special diet! They simply cut back on the foods they were eating and increased their physical activity. It sounds simple. It is the most effective weight loss plan ever devised, and it doesn't cost anything! The only problem with it is that it does take will power and determination to make it work.

I have two male clients that started training at Forever Young about four months before this writing. Both men want to lose weight, put on more muscle, and they are approximately the same age. They are both religious about doing their workouts and they both work out very hard. The results of their labor is that they are both much stronger than when they started, but one man has lost forty pounds and the other has gained six pounds.

The difference between the two is that one man has a wife and family who encourage him to lose weight and they all help him resist temptations. The whole family eats sensibly and it really is a team effort. The other gentleman has a gourmet cook for a wife and the house is filled with all sorts of goodies for the grandchildren, and he can't resist the "goodies"!

Men have little difficulty losing weight. I have no sympathy for the guys that can't get their weight under control. It's just a matter of will power. I have a lot of sympathy for women with the same problem. For the majority of the ladies it's just an uphill battle, and I admire any gal that takes the challenge and wins. They not only naturally carry a higher percentage of fat than men do, but they also face menopause which makes weight loss even more difficult.

Here are a few suggestions to help make the transition from plump to svelte just a little easier. These are life style changes and will work if you stay with them for the rest of your life.

1.   **DO NOT EAT ANYTHING FOR THREE HOURS BEFORE YOU GO TO SLEEP.** For most men and women, just making this simple change in your life style will cause you to lose weight, even if you change nothing else in your eating habits.

2.   **THE EVENING MEAL SHOULD BE THE LIGHTEST MEAL OF THE DAY.** Breakfast and lunch should be the bigger meals. A light snack between breakfast and lunch will keep you from getting a "sugar low". Five small meals through the day is more effective for weight loss than three large ones. More frequent smaller meals are more easily assimilated by the body and will not be stored as fat.

3.   **CALORIES DO COUNT.** If you eat more than you can assimilate, it will be stored as fat. Try to eat foods that are high in volume but low in calories. You cannot eat too many raw or steamed vegetables. Energy requires calories, the more calories you burn, the less calories will be stored as fat. On the other hand, a Big Mac and fries are around four hundred calories more than your allotment for the whole day for most people.

4.   **STARCHY CARBOHYDRATES ARE YOUR WORST ENEMY** if you are on a weight loss plan. Breads and pastas are at the top of the "No-No" list when you are trying to drop the pounds. In all the years my wife and I have been training people, we have never seen anyone drop weight on a high carb plan.

5.   **DO EAT LEAN PROTEIN.** Lean protein would be egg whites, skinless chicken breasts, fish, and turkey. In my experience, the fastest, most effective, way to lose fat is to go on a high protein, low fat, low carbohydrate program. The quantity of protein depends on how hard you are exercising. A beginner should do well on three quarters of a gram of protein per pound of lean body weight. More advanced bodybuilders will eat a minimum of a gram of protein per pound of lean body weight.

While carbs must be kept low, remember you get your first surge of energy from your carbohydrates. There will be a slight loss of energy when you cut back. You may have to experiment to find just what ratio is best for you. It takes at least one hundred grams of carbs to keep your brain functioning properly. So if you start feeling a little slow upstairs, that's a sign you need a few more carbs.

6.   **THE BODY ADAPTS TO A CONTINUOUS PROGRAM.** For example, if you have been restricting your calories to twelve-hundred a day for three months, your metabolism will slow down to adjust to your new eating habits. When your body adapts to a change, you will hit a plateau. The best way to overcome this problem is to shock your body with a new program. There are many ways to change the way you eat and still maintain your weight loss program. Two effective plans I have tried are the Rice Diet and the Variable Calorie Count Diet.

On the Rice Diet you just eat plain rice as often as you like for three days. While rice is a starchy carbohydrate it has no fat. You cannot fancy up the rice. It must be boiled without seasoning, but you can eat as much as you like as often as you like. Believe me in a day or two it will be very difficult to eat too much rice. Most of the people that have tried this diet on my suggestion have lost three pounds in those three days.

Another trick you can use to fool your metabolism is the Variable-Calorie-Count Diet. Let's say you have been on twelve-hundred calories a day for three months, and now nothing is happening with your weight loss. Try this. On the first day of your new plan eat 1800 calories. The second day, you consume 1000 calories, and on the third day you eat 600 calories! Repeat the program for a few weeks and then you can go back to your regular routine. This should break that plateau.

7. SET GOALS. The people who make the most effective weight loss are those with a specific goal in mind. I had one man come into the Studio in February to get in shape for a Fourth of July party that same year. He wowed everyone at the party with his outstanding physique. One of my clients was a world-class swing dance champion. The national championships were in November. He started his training in May. After he won his class that year, he let me know it was his outstanding physique that made him edge out his competitors.

We had a lady working out with us for about a year, who had made so-so results with her training. Her husband was a movie producer who had to represent his company at the Academy Awards Presentation. As soon as she found out she had to go to this prestigious affair, she bore down on her training and diet. Results? She looked stunning in her new gown and new body!

Find an event that is special to you and visualize the way you want to look at that occasion. Keep that vision in front of you continually, and you will reach your goal.

8. KEEP A FOOD JOURNAL. Nothing will keep you on the straight-and-narrow path of dieting better than keeping a Food Journal. With your goal in mind, you record everything you eat. That means everything, even breath mints! To do the Journal properly, you must record the total number of calories in each meal. Then, after the number of calories, calculate the grams of protein, carbohydrates and fats. It sounds like lots of work and at the beginning, it is. After a few weeks, like everything else in life, it will become routine, and you will be amazed at how easy *and effective* the maintenance of the Journal can be.

Karen and I kept a Journal the entire time we participated in bodybuilding competitions. It was just part of our everyday life-style. Though we encourage every client we train to try the Food Journal program, few will put in the effort required to write down everything they eat. *However, all those who keep a Journal reach their weight loss goal on schedule!*

9. USE THE BUDDY SYSTEM. Losing weight is a lonely business. There are constant temptations around you all the time. Find someone to share your goal with you, and the path to success will be much easier. I mentioned the man whose wife and family were pulling with him to reach his goal. That's why he could lose forty pounds so quickly. My wife and I were constantly helping each other to eat properly, so we could get the razor sharp definition that helped us do well in competition.

Very few people can lose weight on their own. That's why all these diet programs are so successful. Save yourself the money a plan would cost you. Get a buddy and have a contest to see who can lose the most weight in a given period of time. Do aerobic work regularly, put the time in with the weights, and you will be amazed at your body's transformation.

10.   DRINK LOTS OF WATER. Nothing helps your body quite as much as pure, plain, unadulterated water. It cleanses your liver, lubricates your joints, and helps pad your body against outside blows. It keeps your skin lubricated, and looking young.

If you are on a high protein diet, you must drink a great deal of water or in all probability you will become constipated. Many advanced bodybuilders drink over a gallon of water a day. It takes at least a couple of liters of water a day for minimum basic requirements for good health. A glass of water before a meal and after a meal will go along way toward limiting the portions of food you can eat at any one meal.

Follow all ten points and in few months you will be delighted with the results you have achieved.

CHAPTER FIVE

AEROBIC WORK
THE FAT BURNER

Oh, the frustrations of burning off that fat. America is plagued right now with an epidemic of obese people. It is not unusual to go to any public gathering and see people who weigh in excess of three hundred pounds. While we were visiting a small town in northern California, my wife and I stopped in at a Denny's restaurant. While there, we saw at least six people that were tremendously obese in that one restaurant!

With all the warnings from T.V. and radio that constantly bombard us with messages of the dangers of being overweight, you have to wonder what compels these people to keep gaining weight? Maybe it's because right after the public service announcement there's a commercial for some fast food product.

One of the most effective ways to combat the fat problem aside from better choices in eating, is with aerobic activity. Any activity that sustains the pulse for a given period of time is an aerobic exercise. Some of the best movements to use for aerobic work are walking, dancing, biking, swimming and rope skipping, just to mention a few.

Covert Bailey, in his book "Fit or Fat", gives a formula to induce the body to get into what he calls the TARGET ZONE. This refers to the ideal pulse rate to use when doing your aerobic exercises.

The formula is based on your maximum heart rate. This heart rate is determined by age. To receive the most effective results for your physical activity, you must keep your pulse within sixty to eighty percent of your maximum heart rate.

Sixty percent of your maximum heart rate, means your body is active enough to be in an aerobic state. You have passed into an anaerobic condition when your pulse has passed eighty percent of your maximum heart rate.

The problem with the formula is it only works if you have a normal pulse rate. If you have a very low pulse or a very high one, another formula has to be followed. In our experiences at our studio few people will take the time to figure out the formula and even less will bother to take their pulse.

A much easier way to determine if you're pulse is in the TARGET ZONE is to follow this simple rule. If your body is warm, you are in an aerobic state. If you can carry on a normal conversation without gasping for more air, you are not overdoing it. It's an easy way to make sure you're making the best use of your time. It may seem silly to be talking to yourself while you're working out, but it's much better than going faster and faster and only defeating your purpose which is to burn off fat!

Always keep in mind that fat burns slowly. When you go too fast your body will need a faster form of fuel to convert to energy. The faster form would be carbohydrates and protein. Carbohydrates burn off rapidly so the body will start using protein as quickly as it can. It gets the protein from your muscle mass. What it's doing is cannibalizing off your muscle to get the energy the body needs to continue in this exercise. So by going fast, you are not only defeating your goal of burning fat, but you are actually reducing your muscle mass!

Most of the literature I have read on using aerobics to get rid of excess weight recommends twenty minutes a day, three days a week. In all the years we have been training people we have never seen anyone lose weight on that amount of work. Five to six days a week of aerobics is the key to success when you are out to burn off that adipose tissue.

The body adapts quickly. I can't emphasize that fact too often. If you work out the same length of time each time you do your aerobic work, your body will adapt. Rather than twenty minutes every workout, try twenty on one day, an hour the next, thirty minutes the following day etc. The more variety in time and exercises, the quicker the results.

For example, when Karen and I were getting ready for a physique competition the aerobics we would do were stationary bike one day, jogging in the park the next day and disco dancing on the following day. In this way the body never knows what's coming up next and can't adapt. That's why we could get our body fat down so low.

Aerobics should be fun--it should something you look forward to doing. There are so many things a person can do for aerobic work, it shouldn't be unpleasant! I have seen a workout session with people waving pie plates while sitting down. Have you ever seen a fat orchestra conductor? Think about it. All they do is wave a baton for hours. It's very aerobic.

If you have avoided Aerobic activity because of joint problems, you should consider working in water. The weightlessness of the body in the water is very sympathetic to the joints. All the "YMCA's" that I have visited have water aerobic classes and they all seem to be very well attended. The point to keep in mind is that any activity that can keep your pulse sustained in the TARGET ZONE for a minimum of twenty minutes is an aerobic activity.

For the more athletic, there are also classes which use boxing movements, Martial Arts movements, Jazzercize classes, step movements and spinning. The list is endless. Find one or two you like follow it faithfully and watch the fat dissolve!

CHAPTER SIX

SENIORS

Aging is not an easy process. If you are going through the many changes that take place during this time, I don't have to tell you the physical difficulties you are experiencing. The joints just don't seem to want to work properly, the fatigue that plagues you never seems to let up and, of course, the skin with the liver spots and the loss of elasticity, all make you wonder why you are being punished so harshly.

Advertisements assure us if you take this pill or use that cream, we can overcome all our health problems, regain the youthful vigor and vitality we all desire plus regain that all important sex drive. I am involved with seniors continually and have yet to find any miracle pill or ointment that has cured a single ailment. The only help I have found so far with most of these problems is exercise and it must be of a resistant type.

It's true aerobic work is necessary and a healthy diet is a must, but lifting weights has to be at the head of the list. Look at almost any person over sixty and you are pretty well going to see the same characteristics. Men will have very skinny arms and legs with a large protruding stomach. Women will have large soft arms and very heavy hips and thighs. Of course, the one thing both men and women have in common with the aging process is the lack of tightness in the skin.

The condition of the skin will really depend on genetic factors. Caucasians will normally have the worst skin problems as far as sagging goes. Blacks, usually, will have the tightest skin. I have body composition tested black people who I believed to be in their twenties and found out they were in their fifties!

If you watch bodybuilding competitions, you will notice the skin condition of the older black athletes is always thicker and tighter than their white counterparts. Even in the young competitors the difference in the skin is quite apparent.

As we age the skin loses it's elasticity. Most seniors are not very active so there is a loss of muscle size. Unfortunately, the skin does not shrink to compensate for this. With a conscientious exercise program the muscle size can be increased to once again fill in that loose skin...depending on how bad the condition has become!

Lifting weights seems to be a miracle cure....or is it? We know muscles respond to exercise at any age, but ligaments and tendons are not so accommodating. That's quite a conundrum when we know that the ligaments and tendons are very much involved with the lifting of weights. These parts are stressed most when using heavy weights. Without increasing the resistance there cannot be any increase in muscle size or strength. Therein lies the problem for the senior bodybuilder. The answer is not to lift heavier weights but to make the weights feel heavier! There are many ways to do this. One way, for example, is in the barbell or machine Bench

Press exercise. For most bodybuilders this exercise demands the heaviest weight for the chest area. If you are doing say three sets of exercises, put the Barbell Bench Press last in the sequence. The two exercises before the Barbell Bench Press might be the Dumbbell Flat Bench Press and the Dumbbell Incline Bench Flys. This will pre-exhaust the chest muscles so that you have to lighten the weight for the Barbell Flat Bench Press. The body doesn't know whether it's lifting fifty or five hundred pounds. It only knows how hard the arms have to push to get it from point "B" to point "C".

If you have gone to failure on the preceding two sets, you will have to use a lighter weight than if you had done the Bench Press at the beginning of the cycle, but the stress on the chest muscles will be as great as it would be with a heavier weight. The same principle would apply if you were doing a heavy Pull-Down for the back or a set of heavy Squats for the thighs.

I recall reading an article written about a discussion between Arnold Schwarzenegger and Frank Zane, two Mr. Olympias. Zane the older of the two said that after fifty, you had to lighten the weights because the body could not take that much stress as it aged. Arnold insisted that was not true, and you must continue to train as heavy as possible at any age. When Arnold turned fifty, his thinking changed!

Another important matter is recovery time. It takes longer for the muscles to recuperate as we age. It took me a long time to accept the fact that exercising three times a week for no more than 1 1/2 hours a day is all I can take. If I exceed that time limit, I'm just too tired to get through the day. The fatigue from over-training can be very demoralizing and is the primary cause for people giving up their physical improvement efforts.

How much is "enough", only you can tell. I've trained some seniors three times a week an hour per session, and they did just fine. Others found three times a week for a half hour workout was best for them. Some, especially at the beginning, found two sessions half an hour long was all they could handle.

The best test is how much you are improving. If your energy is increasing, your strength is going up and you are looking forward to your next workout you are doing everything right. On the other hand, if you are feeling draggy, you have difficulty sleeping and you dread the thought of that next exercise torture, you are doing something wrong, and it's time to rethink the program. People who enjoy a vigorous workout make the most progress and have the most fun at the gym. I know some people find it hard to believe working out can be fun.

The best way to make the exercise sessions more fun and still productive is to have a training partner or a personal trainer. If you can find a companion reasonably close to you in strength, you will be astounded at how fast you will progress. If the partner is much stronger or weaker than you there can be no competition. Who wants to climb an impossible mountain? A few people perhaps, but not very many. On the other hand, if the partner is too weak, he (or she) presents no challenge. You can still have a nice time, but the results in most cases will be nil.

If you can afford it the next best thing to a workout partner is a personal trainer. The trainer can push you to new heights, encouraging you to get that extra repetition out that he knows will give you the desired extra centimeter of muscle mass. If the trainer is good, he is right there all the time so that you can handle more difficult exercises without getting injured or excessively sore from the workout.

The "Golden Years" are not so golden if you are in poor health. An exercise program that includes progressive resistant movements, aerobic activity and a properly balanced nutritional program can make a senior's life useful, productive and...fun!

Muscles respond to exercise at any age, but ligaments and tendons become more brittle with the passing of time. An exercise plan that emphasizes workouts that make the weights seem heavier than they are has it's advantages. Many programs in this manual fool the muscle into thinking the poundages are heavier than they actually are. With this method the muscle will respond with new growth and strength, without stressing vulnerable joints.

Workouts are more fun and far more productive with a workout partner or a personal trainer. It's just too easy to "coast" along with lighter weights if there is no one there to encourage you on to push for that little extra that is so important for gains in size and strength. I know from my own experience without a partner or coach I have to cut my weights almost in half to get through the routine. Ask anyone who has fulfilled some degree of personal excellence and they will all tell you they had a partner or a trainer with them to reach their goal.

CHAPTER SEVEN

TROUBLE SHOOTING

I once complained to Bill Pearl, a many-time Mr. Universe winner, about some aches and pains I had from training. He replied, "You can't train hard at anything without having some pain." Bill was right, of course. The news is filled with reports of injured professional athletes. "No pain no gain" is a familiar phrase to all of us.

Pain is not something most of our clients are anxious to experience. We try our best to plan the workouts so that there is little chance for an injury. We advocate slow and steady progress based on a person's ability and passion. Coaxing a muscle to respond is much better in our opinion than forcing it to grow. With all our caution, there are still some strained muscles.

The trouble with the strain is that the injured muscle cannot be worked until it has improved. Muscles atrophy in seventy-two hours, so you can see if you miss a week, a month or six months you have a problem. Miss a few workouts, and it doesn't take very long to get back to square one. Here, at Forever Young, instead of interrupting our training sessions, we work around the injury.

Most important to prevent injuries is to warm up properly. I always do one or two warm up sets before attempting to work any body part. Take a weight that is relatively easy for the first effort and then do a second set with a weight that is about eighty percent of the poundage you will use for your first real attempt. Proper warm-ups go a long way to prevent any serious training accident.

The most common problem with the lifting of weights seems to be shoulder injuries. Located in the Deltoid is the rotator cuff. This area is where the humerus, clavicle, and scapula bones all converge. It is also where the Pectoralis, Latissimus Dorsi, Trapezius, Biceps, and Triceps all meet, so you can readily see why this area is so vulnerable to injury.

The section commonly affected is the front or anterior Deltoid. This is the pushing part of the Deltoid. The exercise with weights that most often causes the stress in this area is the Bench Press.

The best way to avoid this problem when bench pressing is to lower your arms no lower than perpendicular to your chest. If you already have discomfort with your front Deltoid, discontinue the Bench Press until the injury improves. When you can continue the exercise use the precautions I mentioned earlier. Just because you can't do Bench Presses doesn't mean you have to stop work on your chest. There are many exercises for that area. Experiment until you find something that works without causing discomfort to the Deltoid.

Almost everyone has problems with the lower back. If you are over forty, with few exceptions, you are going to experience discomfort in that area. A lifting belt is a must if you are in this age category. No one strains the lower back more than competitive weight-lifters. I've never seen a lifter in competition or training that wasn't wearing a lifting belt. That should be enough proof of the value of a belt to protect that vulnerable lower back.

Elevating the legs when doing bench work will take pressure off the lower back. Keeping the back flat against the cushions when doing Leg Presses and Sled Squats will prevent injuries to that area. Strict form at all times will help protect this vulnerable area. The thighs should not go below perpendicular to the hip when doing Leg Presses or any form of Squat. Preventing back injuries is easier than trying to cure them.

Knees are something we are cautious about at Forever Young Studio. Three techniques are used here for this problem area. The easiest one to follow is just go very slowly. When you slow the movement down, you have to keep the muscles tight while you execute the movement. Keeping the thigh muscles tight takes pressure off the knee and makes the movement more muscular than skeletal . The poundage has to be lowered when going slow. Lighter weights that feel heavy to the mind can be very effective, and by being lighter they don't put as much stress on the joints.

The next technique involves stutter reps. A stutter repetition is simply a pause for a one, two count during the execution of a movement in an exercise. For example, while lowering the weight in a leg press, just before your legs come to the lowest point in the movement, you pause for a one, two count, and then continue to the low point and finally push back to the starting position.

This makes the move more difficult and you will have to lighten the weight. Remember, the mind doesn't know how much weight you are using. It only knows how difficult it is to move the poundages. If you have to manufacture more muscle to do the job, the body will respond. For years, I used leg wraps to ease the pain in my knees while doing leg exercises. I haven't used leg wraps since I started doing stutter reps, and my legs are as strong now as they were ten years ago!

If one stutter repetition per movement isn't enough to help the situation, add more of these stutters. This way you reduce the stress on the joint or ligament that is causing the problem while still stressing the muscle enough to urge more muscle.

A third method is to simply change the position of your feet. Let's say you are doing the Sled Squat. Your goal is to knock out fifteen repetitions. You start off with your feet straight up and down for the first five reps. Turn your toes out like a waddling duck on the second set of five reps. On the final set of five reps turn your toes in pigeon toe style. This technique of changing the toe position utilizes a variety of thigh muscles to help push the weight, again taking pressure off the knees.

Knee wraps can also help. A wide variety of wraps are available today from the Ace bandage type to sophisticated neoprene wraps with additional supports worked into the fabric. If you are doing record poundages the wraps will help, but if you have to use them continually, reevaluate your training. The knee damage may be structural and need medical attention or you are just training too heavy.

Many of these problems are genetic in origin. I was born with knees that never closed properly. At the fullest point of extension or contraction, the ball joint connection doesn't fit properly. When I was young, the knees were never a problem. In a power lifting contest I needed a three hundred and fifty pound squat to win the competition. It was no problem at twenty. At fifty plus, it was another story. At sixty plus, it's just a distant memory. If the knees were not a genetic problem, however, I could probably still handle that kind of resistance.

The last area we will deal with is the elbow. Prevention is the best cure here. Once an elbow problem hits you, it is very difficult to overcome. The exercises to watch out for are the Lateral Raises for the Deltoids, Curls for the Biceps, and Push-downs for the Triceps. If your form is very strict in the Lateral Raises, you will not be able to handle a lot of weight. You must still try to go to failure, but if your back is held straight, your elbows are in the right position, and you move slowly and deliberately through the movement, you will be amazed at how little resistance is needed to exhaust the muscle.

The same advice applies to the Curl, and Push-Down. A straight back, steady, deliberate movement with the weight, and a full range of movement will prevent this area from becoming inflamed. Go to any gym and watch the gentlemen curling and most of the time they will be handling huge poundages by swinging the barbell to the top of the movement then dropping it and bouncing the weight back up from the bottom with their momentum rather than their biceps. This practice is almost guaranteed to eventually wreck the elbow.

Once the area is injured, it's ice packs first, then elbow wraps. When those don't work it's the doctor for cortisone shots or the acupuncturist and the long needles. All that can be avoided with a sensible program and strict form in all the exercises you perform.

Genetic problems are a different story. A back, knee or elbow problem you were born with requires more research. There is always some exercise that can be performed for the back even though you may have been born with a curvature of the spine. Elbows or knees that can not make a complete range of motion may have to use partial movements to exercise that area. If you can motivate yourself enough, you can overcome any problem.

Libraries are filled with stories of people who overcame incredible handicaps to become Olympic champions. If you want to be really impressed with what can be accomplished with proper motivation, watch any physique show that has a "handicap" category. You will be amazed at the physiques these people develop despite the fact they live in a wheelchair.

Keep in mind always, it is better to prevent an injury than to try to cure it. Always warm up properly before attempting a heavy exercise. The best preventative medicine for resistant type training is strict form. If you must "cheat" to complete a movement, the weight is too heavy.

CHAPTER EIGHT

THE ABDOMINALS

At the top of almost everyone's wish list is the wish for a trim flat muscular waist. The ancient Greeks and Romans stressed strong muscular midsection in all the statues of their men. No modern day bodybuilder, male or female, can do anything in physique competition without outstanding abdominal development.

Not everyone wants to go as far as a real "washboard" effect on their stomach, but almost everyone wants a flat tummy. Whether it's "super abs" or just a smaller belt size, there are some basic premises to follow in any waist reduction program.

The important fact to accept before starting your attack on that flabby middle is that you cannot spot reduce your waist. Most people will lose the adipose tissue (Fat) off their face, shoulders, and legs before it comes off the midsection. Artificial substances such as creams and rubber belts will not help. Their function is to make the exerciser sweat. That they do very well. However, a glass or two of water and the effects of the creams and sweat apparatus are completely lost and the fat will return.

A good abdominal program must start with a good nutritional plan. An effective nutritional program simply means eliminating the foods you know pack on the pounds. Your program must eliminate all fried foods! Restrict all dairy products. Red meats, until you reach your goal, have to be curtailed. If you have a terrible sweet tooth, search for substitutes that are fat free.

Just taking off pounds will not give that youthful athletic figure that most people are looking for. If you go on a well thought out weight loss program, you will lose weight, you will look smaller and you may go down a size or two but you will not necessarily look tighter or more fit...that only comes with exercise.

A few more pointers about the midsection before you start your program. The abdominals really consist of three sections: upper, lower and sides. Each section is important for complete development. The lower abs are the weakest, the sides a little stronger and the upper abs are the strongest. This plan works the weakest muscles first while they are still strong and fresh. Always work the strongest muscles last.

It is essential that while you are doing the ab exercises your lower back is always in contact with the floor. Keeping the back on the floor forces the lower abs to work. If you do not feel the lower abdominals working, it means you are arching your back. If your back is arched, you run the risk of injury.

While doing the exercises that follow, imagine that your midsection is an accordion. Your rib cage is one end of the accordion and your pelvic area is the other end of the instrument. While doing these exercises you are trying to squeeze the ends together so that they meet in the middle. For faster results with your abdominal development squeeze these two ends together as hard as you can.

In movements where you hold your hands behind your head, keep in mind the more you tuck your chin at the top of the movement, the more you will stress the abs. The more you stress your abs, without causing pain, the faster you will get results.

The completion, or the top of the movement, is when you bring the lower rib and the pelvis as close together as you can get them. In each of the movements to follow, when you have squeezed your lower ribs and pelvis as close as you can, hold that position for just a beat. It is the holding or crunching, in that final position that will give you the results you have been striving for. Think always of crunching your abs at the top of the movement and keep that stomach under constant tension through the entire exercise.

Start your routine with an easy number of repetitions for each exercise, then gradually keep adding more repetitions until you get to about twenty reps per exercise. When you can do twenty repetitions on all six exercises go to the next routine. Alternate the routines when you can do twenty reps on all three programs. Remember, the more you vary your exercises, the better the body will respond.

Now the abdominal workout. At our studio we always start the workout with the abdominal routine. We do that for several reasons. One, it is the center of the body which makes it a great way to warm up the muscles. Two, it loosens up the back, avoiding problems in that area when you are exercising. Third, and most important, if you wait till the end of the workout, there's a good chance you will put off the Abs till the next session. If you do the exercises the way I describe them in this booklet, you should see results from your efforts in just a few weeks, especially if you are following a good nutritional program and regular aerobic work.

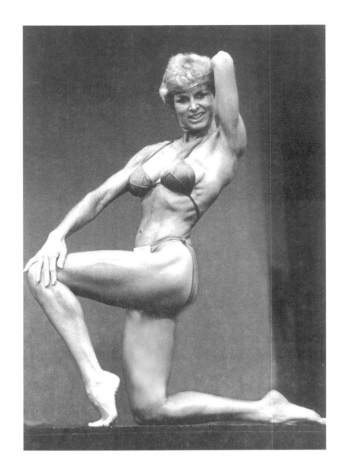

The
TRAINERS

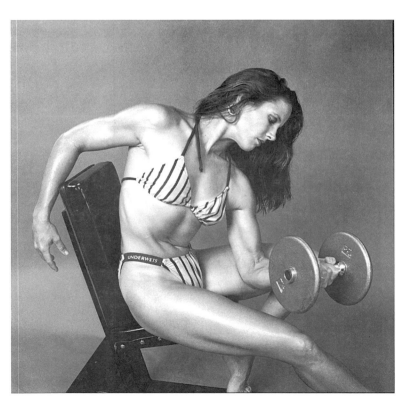

ABDOMINAL ROUTINE
SUPER SIX #1

1. KNEE LIFT CRUNCH
From a lying position, lift both legs twelve to sixteen inches above the floor. Draw one knee to your chest. Curl your torso to the bent leg and grasp the knee with both hands, lifting your forehead to the raised knee. Now alternate your legs with each repetition. Keep the pelvis tilted up through the entire movement. The more you tuck your chin at the top of the movement, the more you will crunch your abdominals.

2. DOUBLE KNEE CRUNCH
Exactly the same as the above, except draw both knees to the chest simultaneously. If there is any lower back discomfort, tilt the pelvis more by raising the legs higher.

3. CROSS LEGGED KNEE CRUNCH
With your legs as illustrated and your hands behind your head, lift your torso as high as you can. Then twist so that opposite elbow and knee touch. Return to original position and repeat the movement. Do one side complete, change leg position, and then do the other side. Don't be disappointed if you can't touch your knee with your elbow at the beginning of your program. With practice and patience you will. You will!

4. BENT LEG CRUNCH
From a lying position, with legs bent as illustrated and feet flat on the floor, simply curl up and crunch, lifting the torso towards the knees.

5. KNEE LIFT TWIST CRUNCH
From a lying position, with hands behind your head, cross your ankles and lift your knees as close to your chest as you can. Twist your knees to the right as far as possible while you twist your elbows to the left and draw your torso and hips together, squeezing the abs tightly. Return your legs to the center position and repeat the same procedure on the other side. As you become more advanced, extend your legs until they are stretched to their maximum length.

6. LEG RAISE REACHING CRUNCH
From a lying position, extend arms fully above your head. Bend both knees and draw them tightly to your chest. While you straighten your legs so that your feet are above your face, reach for the wall in front of you so that your hands reach beyond your legs. The knees do not move. Once the knees are in position, only the hands, feet, and head move. It is important that you raise your head while lifting your arms. To do the exercise correctly, you must see the wall in front of you.

ABDOMINALS
SUPER SIX #1

Start   *Finish*

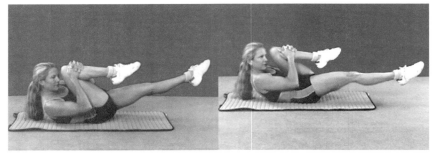

#1 KNEE LIFT CRUNCH

From a lying position, draw one knee to chest, the other extends out above floor. Grasp the bent knee with both hands. Bring forehead to bent knee. Alternate legs with each repetition.

#2 DOUBLE KNEE CRUNCH

Exactly the same as the above except both knees are drawn to the chest at the same time. If there is lower back discomfort, tilt the pelvis more by raising the legs higher to ceiling.

All four lower photos are parts of this one exercise.

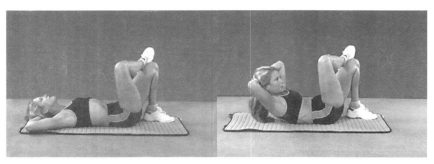
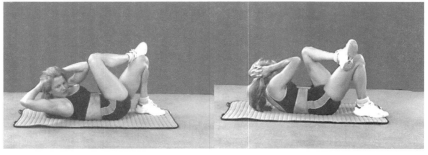

#3 CROSS LEGGED KNEE CRUNCH

Hands behind head, knees bent with right foot on left knee. Lift torso as high as possible, keeping lower back on floor. Then twist left elbow towards right knee and return to start position. Repeat this up, twist, down movement on this one side 20 times before changing to the other side with left foot up.

ABDOMINALS
SUPER SIX #1

Start   *Finish*

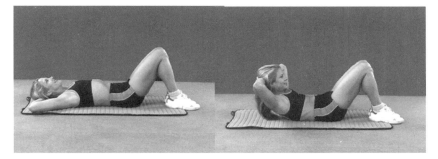

#4 BENT KNEE CRUNCH
From a lying position, with legs bent as shown and feet flat on floor, simply curl up and crunch, lifting the torso but pressing the lower back into floor.

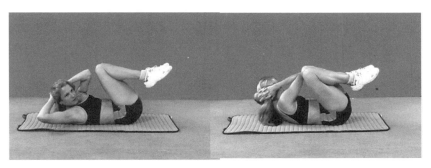

#5 KNEE LIFT TWIST CRUNCH
Hands behind head, knees bent. Twist your knees towards left shoulder while twisting your elbows to right knee. Return knees to center and repeat on other side. As you become more advanced, extend legs as below.

Below is the advanced version of #5 with leg extension in middle of movement

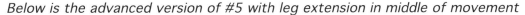

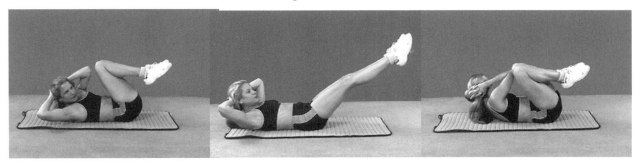

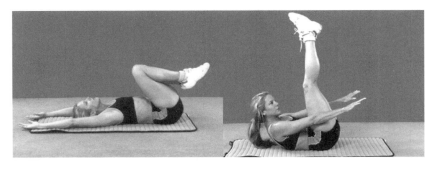

#6 LEG RAISE REACHING CRUNCH
Extend arms fully above head. Bend both knees and draw them close to chest. While you straighten your legs above your face, reach for wall beyond with hands while lifting head and shoulders, squeezing abs tightly. Return to starting position.

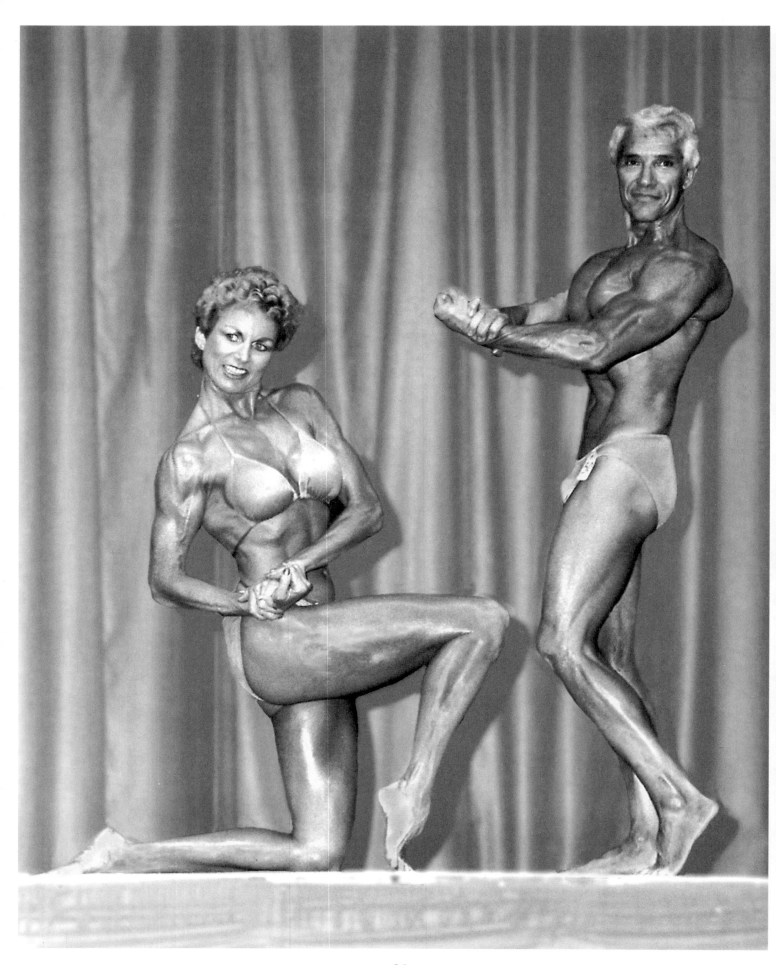

ABDOMINAL ROUTINE
SUPER SIX #2

1. MARCHING STEP
From a lying position, with hands behind your head and legs bent as illustrated, lift your left knee towards your waist and try to touch your right elbow to the raised left knee. Alternate with the opposite elbow and knee.

The resting leg on the floor must have enough weight on it to raise the cheek of the buttocks off the floor slightly.

2. THE ROLL UP
From a lying position, place the hands under the buttocks. Keeping the knees bent as shown, roll the legs up until your knees are at your chest and your feet are over your face.

As your feet come up, your head comes up...always try to squeeze the rib-cage and pelvis together.

3. BICYCLING: SAME ELBOW TO SAME KNEE
From a lying position, with hands behind the head, lift both legs about twelve to sixteen inches above the floor. Bend one leg and draw it towards the waist while reaching forward with the elbow on the same side as the raised knee. Touch elbow to knee. Alternate sides. Be sure to keep both shoulders off the floor.

For maximum results try to touch elbow to knee directly above your belly button.

4. REGULAR CRUNCH: ANKLES CROSSED
From a lying position, with hands behind your head, cross your ankles and hold legs perpendicular to your hips. Lift your torso and try to touch both elbows to both knees. For best results try not to move your legs.

5. BICYCLING: OPPOSITE ELBOW TO OPPOSITE KNEE
From a lying position, with hands laced behind the head, lift both legs twelve to sixteen inches above the floor. Draw one knee towards the waist and try to touch the opposite elbow to the raised knee. Alternate elbow and knee with each repetition. This one is tough! Go easy at first.

6. KICK UP & KICK OUT
From a lying position, with hands under the buttocks, draw both knees to the waist. From this position, kick straight up as high as possible, then draw the knees back to the waist and kick straight out until both legs are fully extended. When you kick out allow the head and torso to lift up and follow the pull of the extended legs. When kicking up try to kick straight up, feet staying over the hips, rather than *...over your head.*

ABDOMINALS
SUPER SIX #2

Start	Middle	Finish

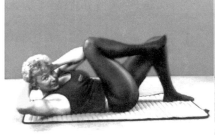 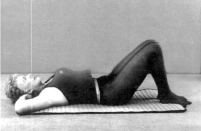 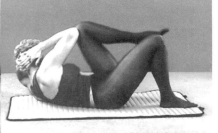

#1 MARCHING STEP *(pictured above)*
Try to touch left elbow to right knee, then down, then right elbow to left knee. One foot always remains on floor with enough pressure on foot to keep pelvis slightly tipped. This prevent the back arching.

Start	Finish

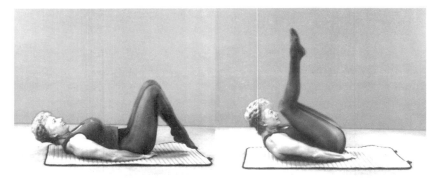

#2 THE ROLL UP
Place hands under buttocks, curl up into ball, knees and shoulders coming together. Keep lower back on floor (pelvis tipped) as feet lower to start position.

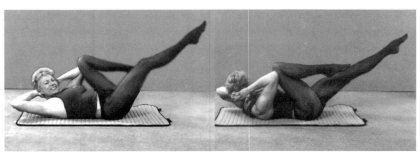

#3 BICYCLING: SAME ELBOW TO SAME KNEE
Lift both legs above floor. Lift your torso and bring left knee to left elbow. Alternate sides, trying to keep both shoulders off floor.

ABDOMINALS
SUPER SIX #2

Start   Finish

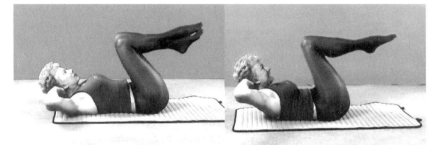

#4 REGULAR CRUNCH: FEET UP
Hands behind head, hold legs perpendicular to hips. Lift torso squeezing ribs & pelvis together.

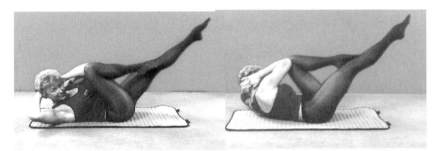

#5 BICYCLING: OPPOSITE ELBOW TO OPPOSITE KNEE
For more advanced version, keep legs closer to floor while maintaining lower back pressing down. If back arches, raise legs back up.

Start   Middle   Finish

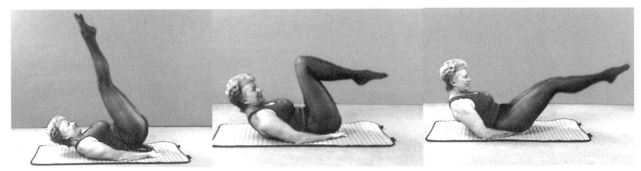

#6 KICK UP & KICK OUT (PICTURED ABOVE)
Hands under buttocks, draw knees to waist. From this position kick straight up. Return to knees bent over waist then kick out towards wall. Allow head and torso to lift up to follow pull of extended legs. You are now in a modified "V" seat position.

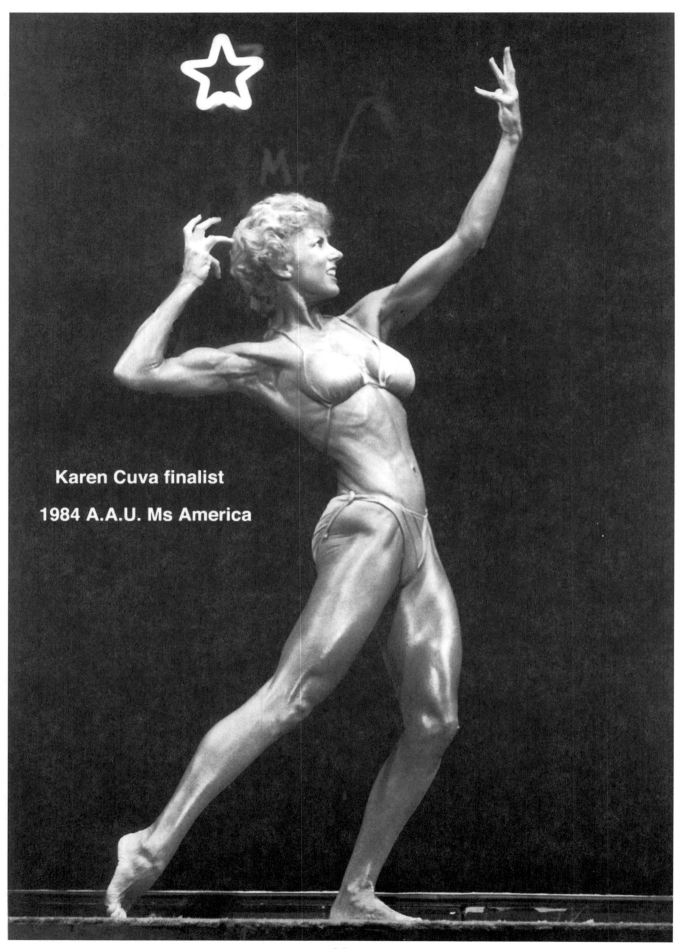

Karen Cuva finalist

1984 A.A.U. Ms America

ABDOMINAL ROUTINE
SUPER SIX # 3

The third routine is the toughest but has only two new exercises. The reason it is so difficult is because of the arrangement of the movements. We are still starting with the weakest muscles, (lower abs), and finishing with the strongest muscle group, (the upper abs).

By sustaining the legs in the air for the first three exercises, the stomach muscles have to work much harder than in the first two routines.

1. BICYCLING: SAME ELBOW TO SAME KNEE
From a lying position, with hands behind the head, lift both legs about twelve to sixteen inches above the floor. Bend one leg and draw it towards the waist while reaching forward with the elbow on the same side as the raised knee. Touch elbow to knee. Alternate sides. Be sure to keep both shoulders off the floor.

For maximum results try to touch elbow to knee directly above your belly button.

2. DOUBLE KNEE IN & OUT CRUNCH
Hands behing head. Squeeze torso and knees together. Extend legs making sure to keep lower back pressed into floor. If back arches up from floor, tilt the pelvis more by raising legs higher.

3. KNEE LIFT TWIST CRUNCH
Hands behind head, knees bent. Twist your knees towards left shoulder while you twist your left elbow to knees. Draw your torso and hips together, squeezing the abs tightly. Return to center and extend legs. Repeat on opposite side.

4. REVERSE BENT KNEE CRUNCH
From a sitting position, with knees bent and both feet on the floor, extend your arms in front of you. Let your torso roll back as far as possible, without collapsing to the floor. Now raise your upper body about two or three inches. You should raise your torso just high enough to feel the abs straining, but not high enough for them to relax. The abdominals must stay tensed through the entire range of the exercise.

5. BICYCLING: OPPOSITE ELBOW TO OPPOSITE KNEE
From a lying position, with hands behind the head, lift both legs twelve to sixteen inches above the floor. Draw one knee towards the waist and try to touch the opposite elbow to the raised knee. Alternate elbow and knee with each repetition. This one is tough! Go easy at first.

6. TOE TOUCH CRUNCH
From a lying position, lift both legs up till your feet are directly over your belly button. Reach up with your arms and try to touch your toes. Then lower your shoulders and repeat the motion. If you can't touch your toes at first, don't give up. If you are persistent and regular with your training, you will be amazed at how flexible you will become!

ABDOMINALS
SUPER SIX #3

Start   Finish

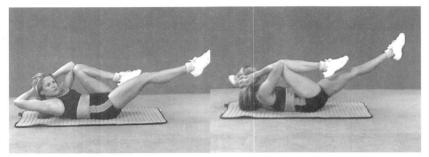

#1 BICYCLE LEGS: SAME ELBOW TO SAME KNEE
Hands behind head, lift both legs off floor. Bend left leg towards waist while reaching left elbow to same knee. Alternate sides. Be sure to keep both shoulders off the floor.

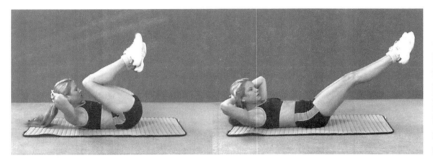

#2 DOUBLE KNEE IN & OUT CRUNCH
Hands behind head. Squeeze torso and knees together. Extend legs making sure to keep lower back pressed into floor. If back arches up from floor, tilt the pelvis more by raising legs higher.

All four pictures below illustrate parts of this one exercise

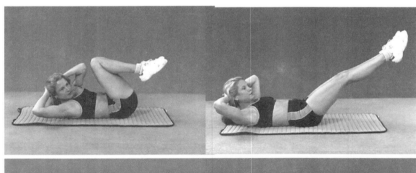

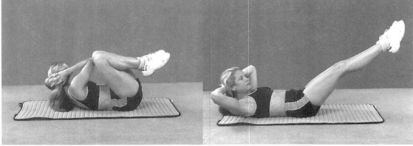

#3 KNEE LIFT TWIST CRUNCH
Hands behind head, knees bent. Twist your knee towards left shoulder while you twist your left elbow to knees. Draw your torso and hips together, squeezing the abs tightly. Return to center and extend the legs. Repeat on opposite side

ABDOMINALS
SUPER SIX #3

Start   Finish

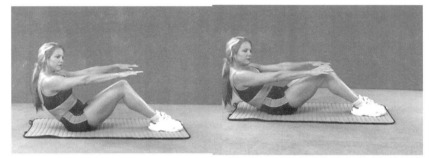

#4 REVERSE BENT KNEE CRUNCH

From a sitting position, with knees bent and both feet on the floor, extend your arms in front of you. Let your torso roll back by tilting the pelvis as far as possible without collapsing to the floor or feet coming up. Now raise your upper body about three or four inches and repeat up & down.

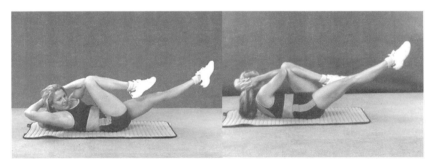

#5 BICYCLE LEGS: ELBOW TO OPPOSITE KNEE

Hands behind head, lift both legs off floor. Bend left leg towards chest while reaching right elbow to touch knee. Alternate sides. Be sure to keep both shoulders off the floor.

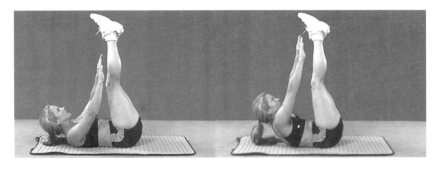

#6 TOE TOUCH CRUNCH

Lift both legs straight up as pictured. Reach up with your arms and try to touch your toes. Then lower your shoulders and repeat motion.

CHAPTER NINE

THE CHEST
HELPFUL HINTS

I believe most of us think of the pectoral muscles when we think of the chest. Everyone would like to have great looking "Pecs" but there is more to the chest than just the pectorals. A great part of the chest size is in the rib cage. The serratus magnus, (those rib like muscles that run down the sides of the chest) add a great deal of aesthetic beauty to the total picture of the chest.

Heavy leg work that forces you to breath deeply is the most effective way to increase the size of the ribcage. Any form of exercises that use the legs, followed by a deep breathing exercise will force the ribcage to grow. There are recorded cases of men putting one or two inches on their chests after only one month of heavy Squats followed by Straight Arm Pullovers. For this method to be effective, you must be breathing very hard, so keep the repetitions high. If you want a larger chest, try those exercises for a month.

The function of the pectorals is to push things away from the body and to help cross the arms. Try to visualize the muscles while you are doing the exercise. It is easy for the arms to do all the work rather than the chest muscles. The mind goes to the familiar. It will want to use the arms. You will have to train your mind to use those chest muscles.

A simple way to isolate the pectoral muscles is to extend your arms in front of your chest. Clasp your hands together and then push the hands against each other. You should feel the muscles of the chest contract. This contraction of the pectorals you feel is the sensation you are seeking when doing your chest exercises.

When doing your Bench Presses, keep your shoulder blades pressed together. By pressing the shoulder blades in this manner you force the shoulders to stay pressed deeply into the bench. This procedure will help you lift the maximum poundages you are capable of without damaging the front deltoid.

Fly movements are isolation exercises for the pectorals. In these flying movements, the elbows are kept bent. When the weight descends, try to get as much stretch as you can without stressing the Deltoids. When you return the weight to the starting position think of wrapping your arms around a great big tree trunk. This will force you to lift your arms up wider and higher than the position you lowered the dumbbells. Lifting your arms in this manner forces the pectorals to do the work instead of all the supporting muscles. Visualizing the muscle while you're doing the exercise is a great help.

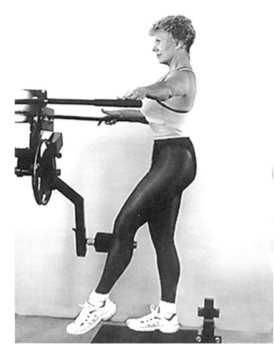

Karen Cuva age 54

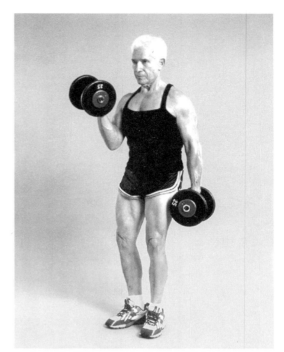

Frank Cuva age 69

Dennis Zisfain age 44

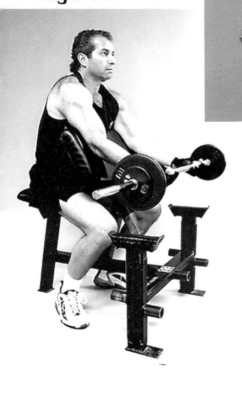

Bob Thompson age 55

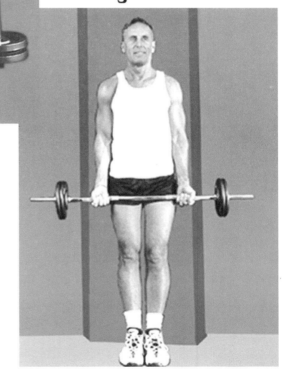

Gail Hazard age 55

CHEST
ON MACHINES

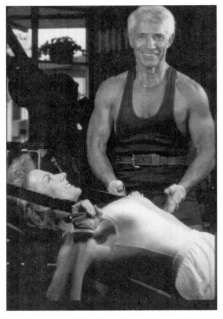 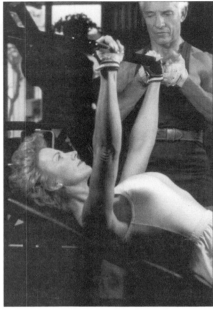

MACHINE INCLINE BENCH PRESS

It's always best to have a training partner if possible. With machines, if you are in the proper position, it is almost impossible to do the exercise incorrectly.

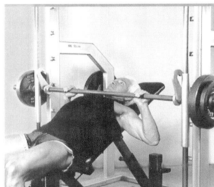 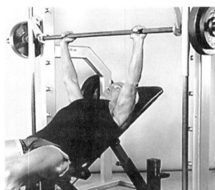

SMITH INCLINE BENCH PRESS

Incline work involves the upper pectoral muscles. The advantage of the Smith Machine is, if you get stuck because the weight is too heavy, you just flip your wrist and the bar settles on the safety hooks. This is a great feature if you do not have a training partner.

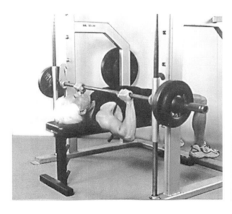 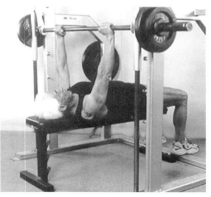

SMITH FLAT BENCH PRESS

Place the bar well back on the thick section of your hand. Lift the bar off the rack. Lower the weight to the chest and then push back to the starting position.

CHEST
FLAT BENCH

Start   *Finish*

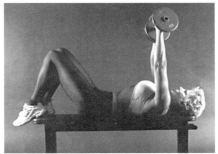 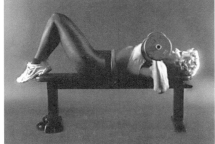

FLAT DMB PRESS
Just press up and together then lower weights, keeping elbows wide and back towards ears rather than stomach to isolate the Pectorals.

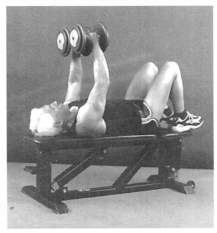 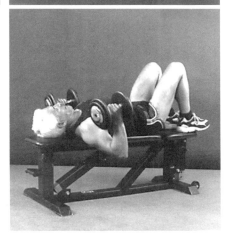

PALMS IN DMB PRESS
Same as above except palms are facing each other through entire movement.

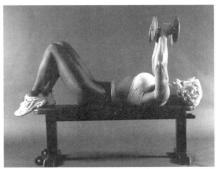 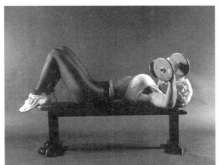

FLAT DMB FLYS
Elbows slightly bent, palms facing each other. Lower arms to your sides then reach out and up with your hands as if reaching around a large tree trunk.

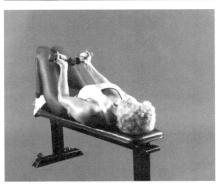 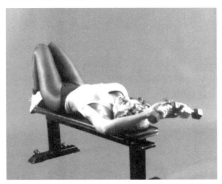

FLAT DMB ROUND THE WORLD
Move the arms in a half circular motion from top to bottom of movement.

CHEST
INCLINE BENCH WORK

Start &Finish   Middle

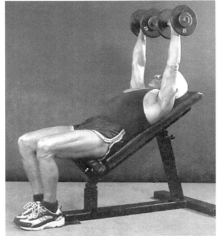
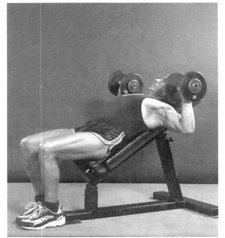

INCLINE DMB PRESS
To get maximum benefit to Pectoral muscles, keep the elbows well back toward the ears as you raise and lower the weight.

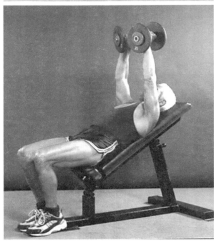
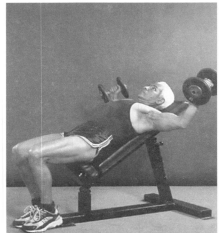

INCLINE DMB FLY
Palms facing each other, lower Dmbs with elbows well bent and wide. Open the arms as you raise the weight, as if you were putting your arms around a huge tree trunk.

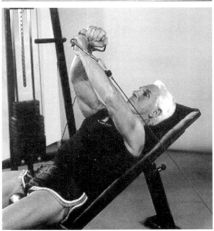
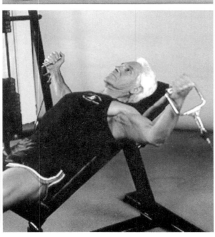

CABLE INCLINE FLY
It is important in this exercise to always keep the elbow in line with your wrist. If the elbow is twisted towards the waist, there is a chance you can lose control of the weight.

CHEST
WITH CROSS-OVER CABLES

Start & Finish   *Middle*

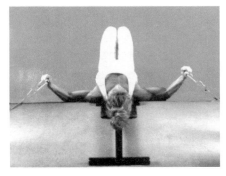 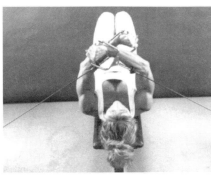

X-OVER FLAT FLYS
Keep elbows slightly bent through entire movement.

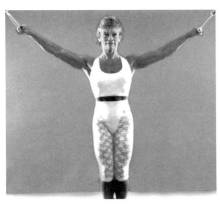 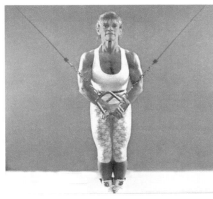

X-OVER STANDING FLYS
As you pull the handles down, lean forward and try to contract the Pectoral muscles.

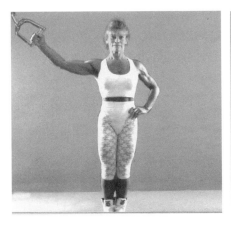 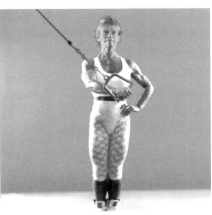

X-OVER 1-ARM FLYS
Contract the Pectorals as the handles reach the end of the movement.

CHEST
DIPS

Start & Finish *Middle*

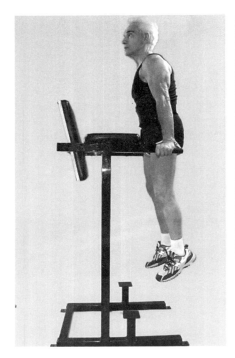 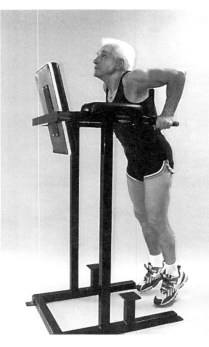

PARALLEL DIPS
Elbows wide for best Pectoral development. Keep the elbows wide and away from the torso.

If elbows are kept close to the body the Triceps become the primary muscle group.

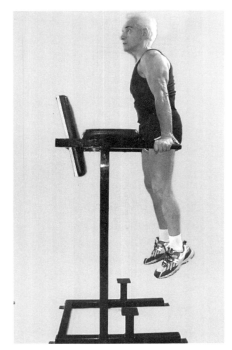 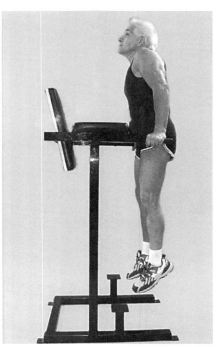

PARRILLO DIPS
The arms do not bend in this exercise. Pause at the top and bottom of movement.

CHEST
DECLINE BENCH WORK

Start & Finish	Middle

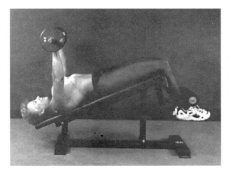 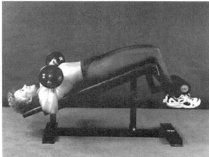

DECLINE BBL BENCH PRESS
Same as flat bench press except this press works the lower pectorals. You can usually use more weight on the decline than on the flat or incline benches.

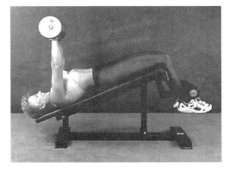 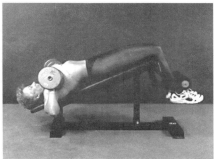

DECLINE DMB BENCH PRESS
Think of pressing the weight in the direction of your waist.

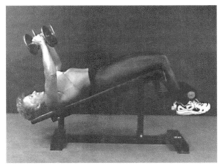 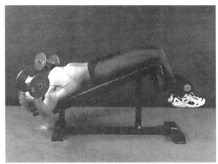

DECLINE DMB FLYS
By changing equipment you use different muscle fibers and it keeps the workouts more interesting.

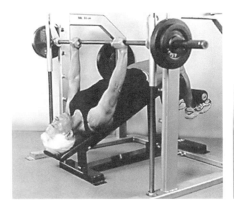 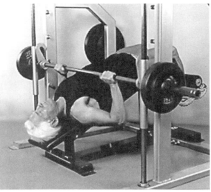

SMITH DECLINE BENCH PRESS
Lower the bar to the sternum and then push back to starting position

CHEST

Start & Finish   *Middle*

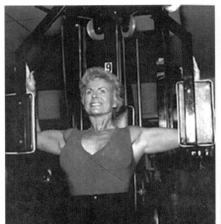 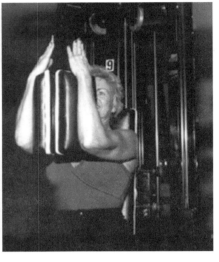

PEC DECK
Elbow straight out in line with shoulders. Open and close handles pushing with the elbows. Focus on squeezing the chest.

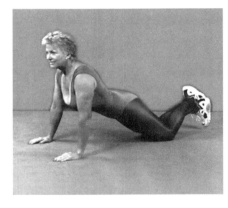 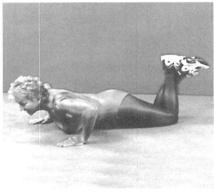

PUSH UPS

Modified, beginner position

Raise & Lower from knees.

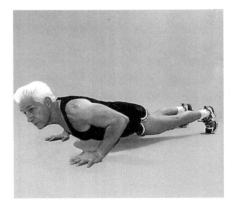 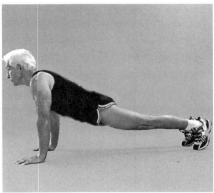

Advanced Position
Raise & Lower from toes.

Keep hands more than shoulder width. Touch chest to floor with each repetition.

CHEST
COMBINATION EXERCISES

DMB PULLOVER & PRESS COMBINATION

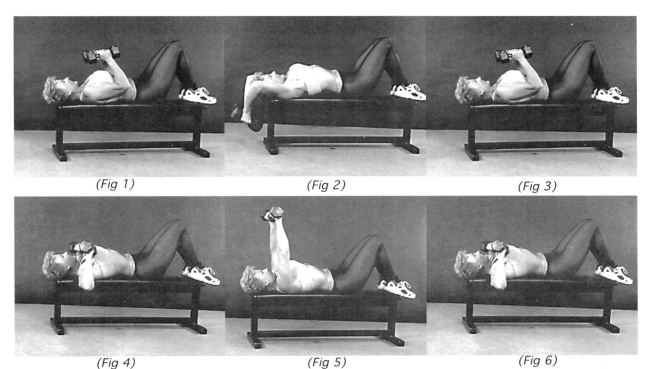

(Fig 1)   (Fig 2)   (Fig 3)

(Fig 4)   (Fig 5)   (Fig 6)

Use two dumbbells. Keep elbows in during start of exercise *(Fig 1)*, lower weights over and past face towards floor as low as possible without shoulder discomfort *(Fig 2)*. Then pull the weights back to starting position *(Fig 3)*. Bring elbows out to sides and proceed to press straight up *(Fig 4 & 5)*, then down (Fig 6), and return to starting position.

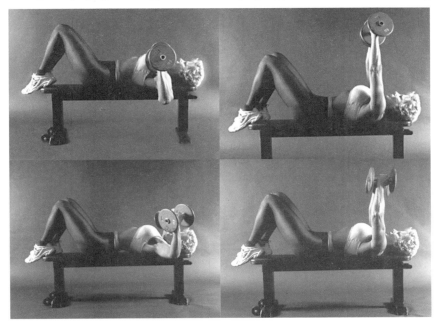

DMB PRESS & FLY COMBINATION

Lower weights with elbows back towards ears. Press straight up. Twist palms to face each other with elbows slightly bent, lowering dumbbells wide to a comfortable stretch. When returning to start position, reach out and up as if putting your arms around a huge tree trunk. Rotate palms to start again.

CHAPTER TEN

THE BACK
HELPFUL HINTS

When we talk about the back, we are really talking about the Trapezius, Latissimus Dorsi, and the Spinal Erectors muscles. The Cobra like shape advanced bodybuilders display when they show off their back, consists of this group of muscles. Each group requires a distinct approach in your training, but the results are well worth the effort.

The Trapezius runs from the top of the neck to the tip of the shoulders to the middle of the back forming a diamond shape. It is a muscle we use constantly. Every time you raise your arms or lift an object, the Trapezius is used. This constant use makes it a very difficult muscle group to develop so we advocate an intense program if you want results. On most of the exercises we do for this area of the back we use high repetitions, especially for the Shoulder Shrugs.

The Latissimus Dorsi or "Lats" are the muscles that give the torso that beautiful taper from shoulder to waist that only gymnasts and bodybuilders possess. This is a relatively easy area to develop, if you can isolate the muscle. The trick to exercising this body part is using the back and not the arms to move the weight. The mind goes to the familiar, so it will want to use your arms to do the pulling.

The best way I have found to train the mind to accept the back as the source of power in doing Lat work, is to contract the back muscles before bending my arms to make that initial pull. Extend your arms to their maximum limit before starting to pull on the weight. Then draw your shoulder blades back and down before bending your arms. Once the weight has started, you then can bend the arms to complete the move.

If you still have difficulty feeling the Lats initiate the movement, try this exercise. The Pull-Down movements are just an easier way to do a pull-up. Few people today can do a good pull-up to the chinning bar without help of some kind. With the Pull-Down equipment you can use less than bodyweight to get benefit from the exercise. To get the feel of this movement, grasp a chinning bar with your hands shoulder-width apart. Now pull your body toward the bar without bending your arms. Your feet can stay on the ground while you are pulling your torso toward the chinning bar. Throw your head back as far as possible while you continue pulling on the bar. Remember do not bend your arms! You will feel your Lats contract, and this is the feeling you want to achieve when performing any Lat exercise.

The lower part of the Lat is a more difficult area to isolate. Normally, only advanced bodybuilders develop these muscles so that they are easily visible. When the lower Lat is highly developed, the lower back has a "Christmas Tree" like look when the back muscles are flexed. Look at any photos from a Mr. Olympia contest and you can see what I'm describing here.

To hit this area in the Pull down, pull the weight to your sternum on the downward movement. Keep your elbows tight against your sides when you reach the bottom part of the exercise. You should feel those lower back muscles contract at that point. Try to visualize the muscles working. Using this technique should show results in a short time.

The Spinal Erectors complete the back area. These are the muscles that flank the spine. For most of us this is a vulnerable spot. When performing Dead Lifts or Good Morning exercises keep your back flat. You can do this by keeping eye contact with yourself in the mirror. Problems with the back usually happen when the back is rounded. Stiff-Legged Dead Lifts are an exceptionally good exercise for developing the buttocks and hamstring muscles, but should only be performed if your back is in exceptionally good condition. This is an important group of muscles to work. They must be worked with caution to be productive.

REMEMBER STRICT FORM IS THE WAY TO PREVENT INJURIES!

BACK
PULL-DOWNS

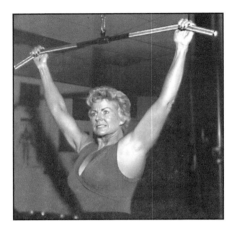

Start & Finish
In overhead position
go to full arm extension.

Middle Position Shown Below

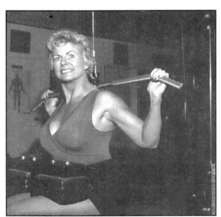 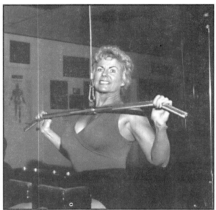

WIDE GRIP PULL-DOWN

BACK *(left)*

FRONT *(right)*

Arching the back and pulling
the bar until it touches the
back or chest works the
lower part of the Latissimus
Dorsi.

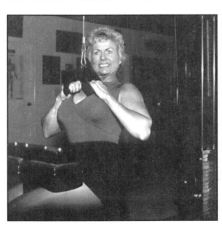 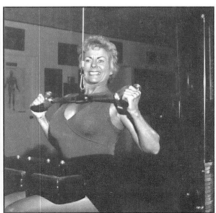

CLOSE GRIP *(left)*

ROUND GRIP *(right)*

Whenever you change the
handles, you work different
fibers of the same muscle

BACK
1-ARM EXERCISES

Start & Finish　　　　*Middle*

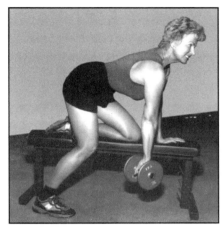 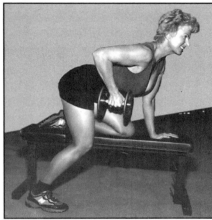

1-ARM DMB ROW
Try to draw the weight to the body with the back muscle. Use the arms as little as possible.

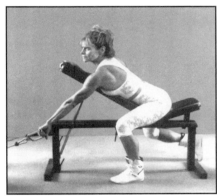 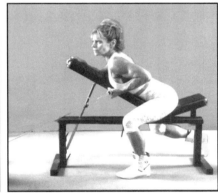

CABLE INCLINE 1-ARM LOW PULL
Bring the handle to the chest, (keeping the arm straight as long as possible before bending the elbow), to complete the exercise.

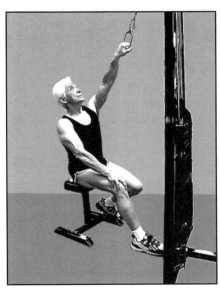 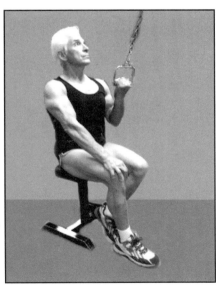

CABLE 1-ARM HIGH PULL-DOWN
Note the position of the hands at the start and finish of exercise

BACK

Start & Finish   Middle

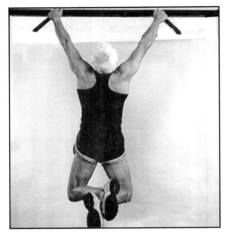 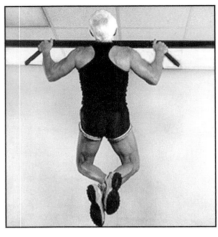

WIDE GRIP PULLUPS
Start the movement with the body fully lowered and arms straight, then pull up until your chin is above the bar.

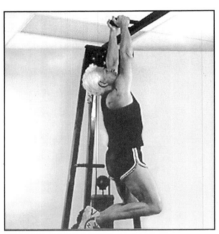 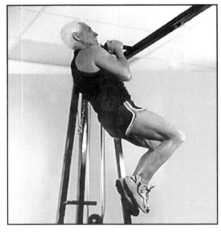

CLOSE GRIP PULLUPS
Start from the fully lowered position and pull yourself as high as you can. If you can pull to the Sternum, you will work the lower part of the Latissimus Dorsi, a very difficult area to exercise.

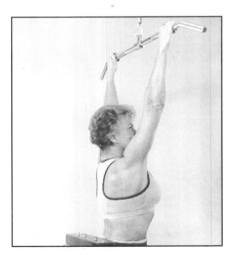 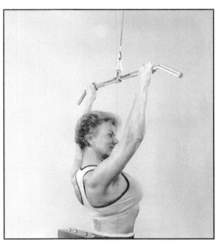

PULL-DOWN SHRUGS
This exercise is used to pre-exhaust the "Lats". With most people, the armsbecome tired before the Lats are affected. With arms straight, pull the weight down as far as you can, then squeeze the shoulder blades to-gether. If done correctly, the movement will look like a "J". After forming the "J", reverse the motion and return to start position.

BACK
ROWS

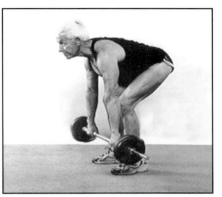

Shown with BBL in Start & Finish Positions

BENT OVER ROW
Keep knees bent and the back in a flat position. The best way to flatten the back is to look straight ahead.

Middle Position

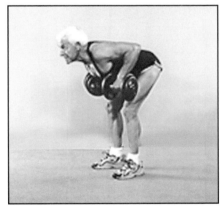

Shown With DumbBells

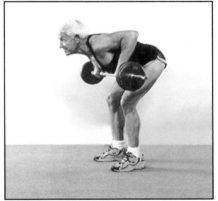

Shown With BarBell

Pull the weight to the chest and then lower to starting position. The hands are held together at chest level as illustrated.

Start

Finish

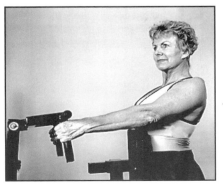

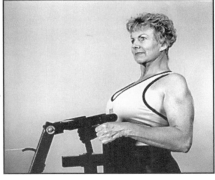

SEATED ROW
Draw the handles to your chest by pulling the shoulder blades together before you bend your arms. For best results keep the chest pressed against the pad through out the entire movement.

BACK
HIGH BENCH ROWS

Start & Finish   *Middle*

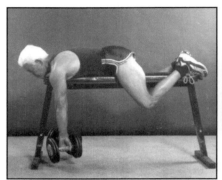 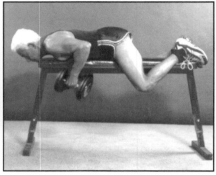

HIGH BENCH
DMB ROWS
Draw the shoulders back
before bending the arms
for the best results.
Think of rowing a boat.

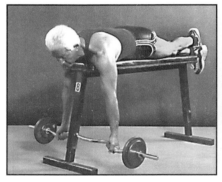 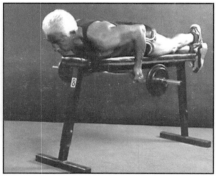

HIGH BENCH BBL
REVERSE GRIP ROW
Use underhand grip and
pull bar towards the
middle of your waist.

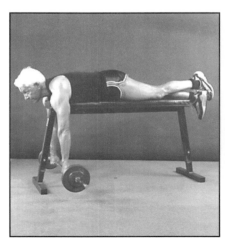 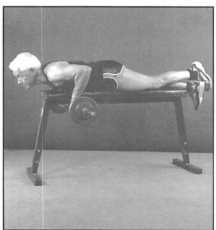

HIGH BENCH BBL
REGULAR GRIP ROW
Use overhand grip and pull
the weight to the chest.

BACK

Start & Finish   Middle

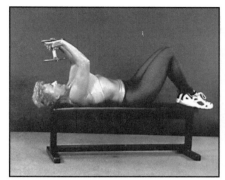 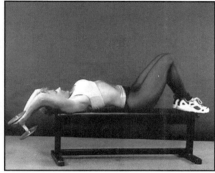

BENT ARM PULLOVER
With elbows bent, hold Dmb directly over face. Move weight over head and down towards floor keeping elbows bent. Repeat movement.

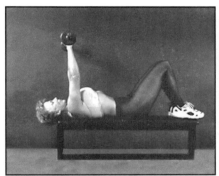 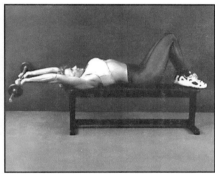

STRAIGHT ARM PULLOVER
Hold BBL straight up over shoulders. Keeping arms straight, lower bar as close to floor as comfortably possible. Raise to starting position and repeat.

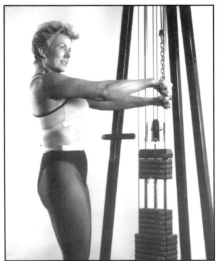 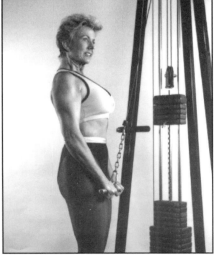

STRAIGHT ARM PUSHDOWN
With arms straight at shoulder level, push the weight down to your thighs as you thrust your pelvis forward. If you are doing the exercise correctly, you will feel it in the lower "Lats".

BACK
LOW BACK

Start & Finish   Middle

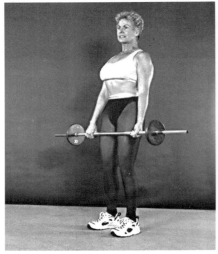 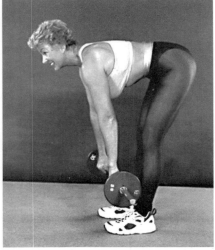

STRAIGHT LEG DEAD LIFT
Keep looking straight ahead to keep back in the strongest position possible. Keep shoulders back at top of movement.

Not for people with low back problems!

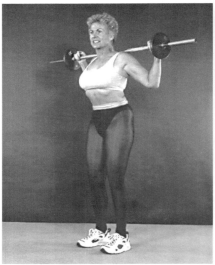 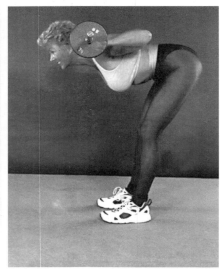

GOOD MORNINGS
Keep knees slightly bent. Same as shown above.

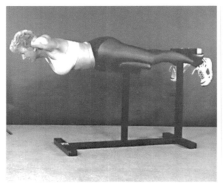 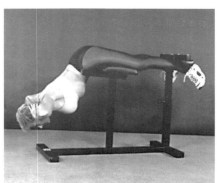

HYPEREXTENSIONS
When first attempting this exercise, keep hands behind lower back until movement is easy.

BACK
BACK & LEGS

Start & Finish

Middle

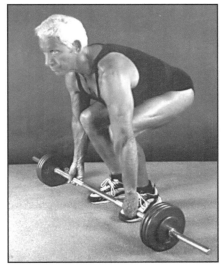 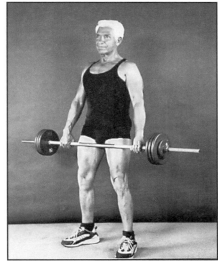

BENT KNEE DEAD LIFT
Squat with BBL in hands. Head up, back straight, hips lower than shoulders. Straighten to upright position and return to floor.

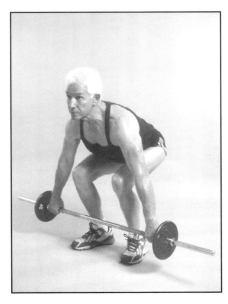 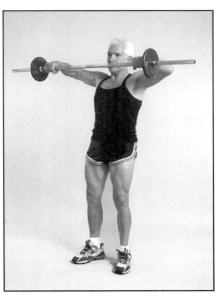

HIGH PULL UP
Wide grip, hands wide. Lift keeping BBL forward of body and elbows up.

TRAPEZIUS
SHRUGS

Start & Finish   *Middle*

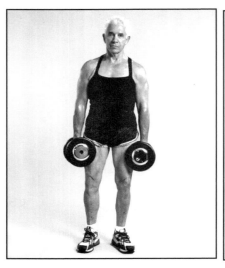 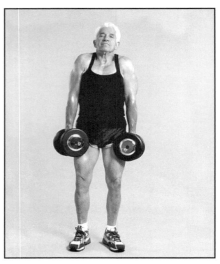

DMB SHRUGS
On all Shrugs the arms must just hang limp. Let the "Traps" do the work. Do not bend the elbow. Just raise & lower shoulders.

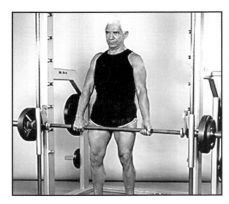 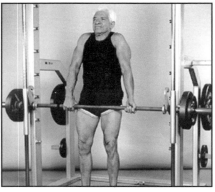

SMITH MACHINE SHRUGS

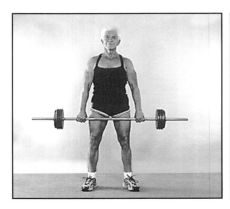 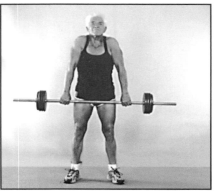

BBL SHRUGS
Changing the equipment works different muscle fibers and keeps the workouts fun!

BACK, LEGS & SHOULDERS COMBINATION
CLEANS

Start   *Finish*

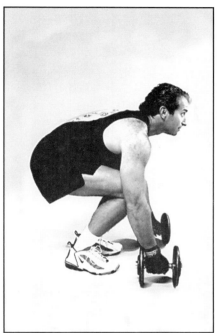 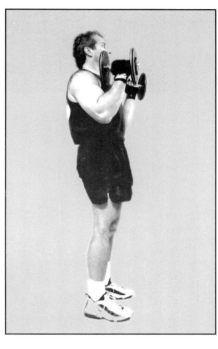

DMB CLEANS
One quick movement from floor to shoulder, then repeat.

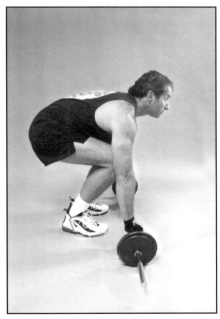 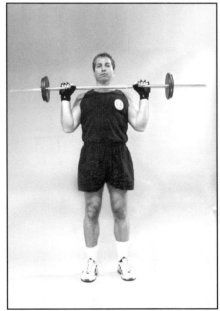

BBL CLEANS
Same as Above

Look straight ahead as you pull and lower the weight in all cleaning movements.
Keep the weights close to the body as you pull the bar to your shoulders.
Keep back flat at all times.

BACK, LEGS & SHOULDERS COMBINATION

BBL CLEAN & PRESS

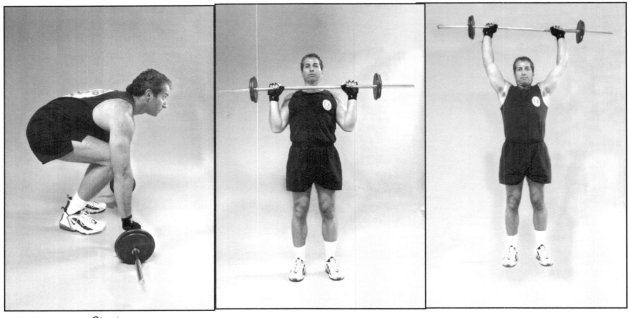

Start   *Middle*   *Finish*

Pull weight to chest in one movement, keeping the bar close to the body. Without any body movement lift the weight from the shoulders to full arms length overhead. Drop the weight to the shoulders, then lower weight to floor, bending knees.

DMB CLEAN & PRESS

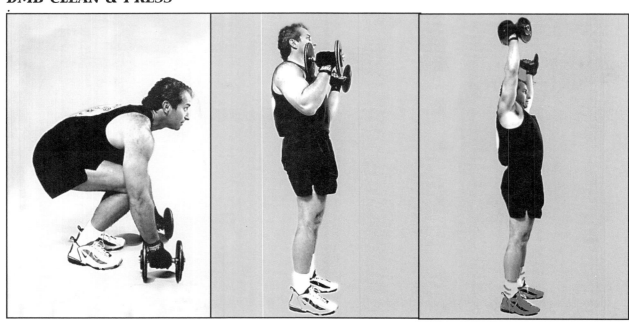

Every time you change the equipment for the same exercise, you use different muscle fibers.

CHAPTER ELEVEN

THE LEGS
HELPFUL HINTS

The secret to success in bodybuilding and an active senior life is a consistent and intelligent leg program. Working the thighs with enthusiasm benefits the entire muscular system. When you move those heavy weights with your thighs, you stimulate the growth hormone. This hormone stimulates muscle growth through the entire body. The harder you push those thighs; the more your whole body benefits from the effort.

With most people the thighs are one of the easier muscle groups to respond to resistant type exercises. If you're pushing to the limit in your leg program, you should see results within a month or two. The trick, as we get a little older, is to push to the limit without ruining our knees, hips or lower back. If you start your program with these problems (stiff or sore knees, hips, or lower back), you must be very careful in your efforts so as not to worsen your condition.

When performing Squats or the Leg Press on the machines, if you put your feet as high on the platform as you can, you take pressure off your knees. Doing the movements slowly, so that the muscles of the thighs stay tight, will also help with this problem. Here's another trick to help the knees. In the negative part of the exercise (that's the part when your legs are going to the lowest part of the movement); just before you're thighs get to the bottom, take a brief pause or stutter then complete the movement and start pushing back to the top. This will relieve even more pressure from the knees.

You will not see any Squats in this program with a barbell sitting across the shoulders. Heavy Squats are fine for the very young, but this manual was written for the more mature bodybuilder. I'm sure there are many senior citizens that can do the regular squat, but most of us will have problems with the lower back if we do this exercise with the bar across your trapezius muscles. The Sled Squat, the Hack Squat and the Leg Press are much safer and every bit as effective for our purposes.

To keep the pressure on the legs and not the lower back, keep two things in mind. First, it is unnecessary to bend or lower the thighs more than ninety degrees. As long as your thigh is perpendicular to your hip, you have gone deep enough in this movement. Second, by pressing your lower back and buttocks deep into the pad you will avoid injuries to this area. Strict form is the best way to avoid training problems.

The calves are, by most people's standard, the toughest muscle in the body to develop. If you want any success at all in this area, you must be merciless in your training. If you can complete a calf exercise and then walk normally after the set, you haven't pushed hard enough! At our training studio we recommend high repetitions, twenty or thirty per set. We encourage our clients to use full extension and full contraction on each repetition. That means stretch as low as you can on the bottom of the movement and squeeze as much as possible at the top of the exercise. Remember, even if you do not increase the size of your calves, the important thing is that you will walk, run, climb, swim and dance better and more easily with regular calf work.

LEGS
ON MACHINES

Start & Finish   *Middle*

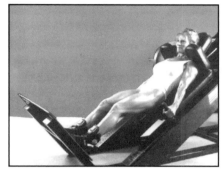
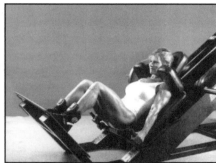

HACK SQUAT
Press back into support and lower body until thighs are parallel to the platform, then push back to the starting position.

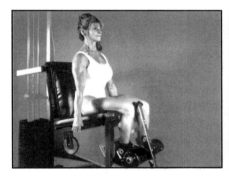
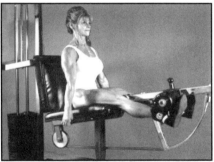

LEG EXTENSION
Lean back into seat. Keep feet flexed and toes turned in as you raise and lower weight.

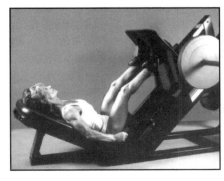
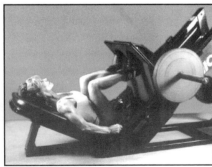

LEG PRESS
Keep hips pressed down into machine while bending knees. Do not allow hips to roll up. Lower weight until the thighs are perpendicular to the hips then thrust legs back to starting position.

LEGS
ON MACHINES

Start & Finish   Middle

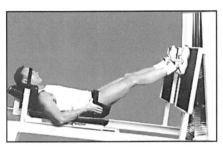 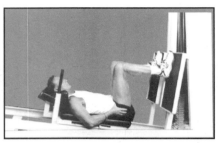

SLED SQUAT
Keep back pressed into pad. Bend knees until perpendicular to hip, then straighten legs keeping knees slightly bent at top.

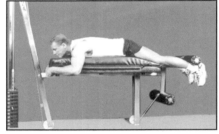 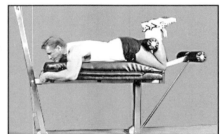

LYING LEG CURL
Keep pelvis tight against pad while bringing feet up.

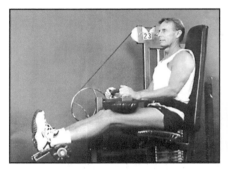 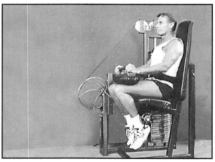

SEATED LEG CURL
Pull back strong, then release with a controlled slow movement. Upper body remains stationary.

(Shown leaning back)

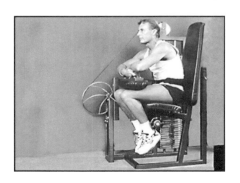

Alternate Position:
Seated Leg Curl leaning forward. This position is sometimes easier on lower back.

LEGS

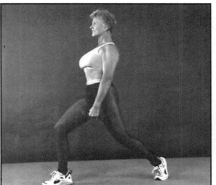 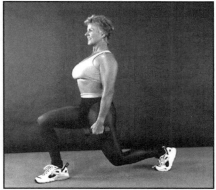

LUNGE
Keep body centered and upright between the front & back legs. Do not let forward knee extend over toe area. Knee must stay over ankle.

You may hold Dmbs in hands or a BBL behind the neck. Raise & lower body as shown. Alternate Legs.

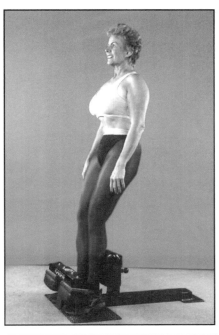 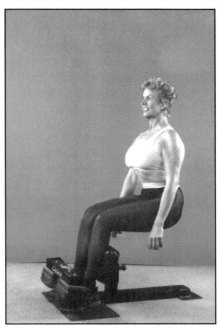

SISSY SQUAT
In this squat the more you lean back the more effective the movement.

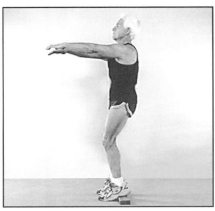 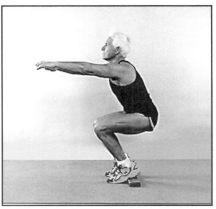

REGULAR SQUAT
Legs comfortably apart, lower your body until your thighs are perpendicular to your hips, and then return to starting position. A block under the heels will help maintain your balance and keep the back straight. If additional resistance is desired, hold a dumbbell in each hand or place a barbell across the shoulders.

LEGS
SIDE LEG MACHINE

Start   *Finish*

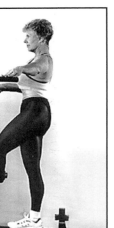 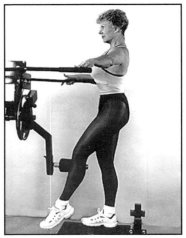

SIDE LEG MACHINE IN
The supporting leg faces forward with the knee slightly bent. Keep the hips stationary during movement so as not to strain the lower back. Draw the weight across to the front of supporting leg then return to out position. Do the exercise slowly to really feel the muscle. This does not require power.

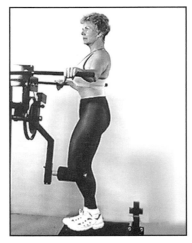 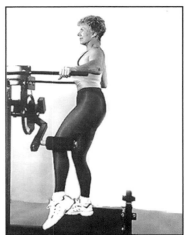

SIDE LEG MACHINE OUT
Similar to inner thigh above, except the pad is on the outside of leg. Do not swing the leg. Maximum benefit comes with slow controlled movement.

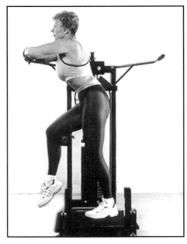 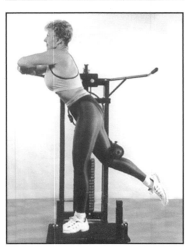

SIDE LEG MACHINE BACK
Kick leg back, squeeze the buttocks in the back position and hold for a beat. Keep the torso upright while completing movement.

LEGS & CALVES

Start	Finish

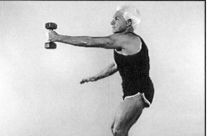 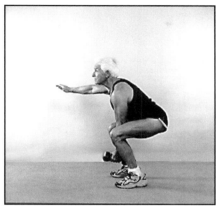

DMB SWING
Excellent warm up for legs. Look straight ahead to keep the back flat. Toss DMB from hand to hand at shoulder height between each squat.

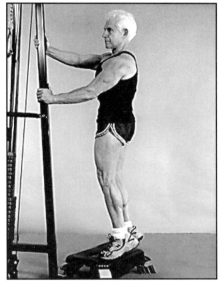 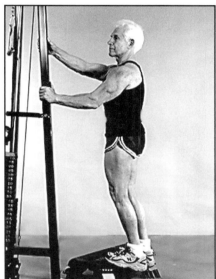

STANDING CALF RAISE BOTH LEGS
Stand on top of a structure that allows you to lower your heels to the maximum stretch. Rise as high as possible on toes, then lower your heels to complete the movement. If additional resistance is desired, hold a dumbbell in one hand.

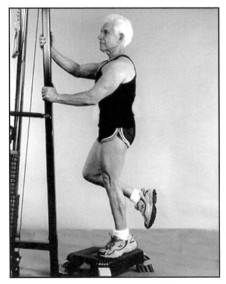 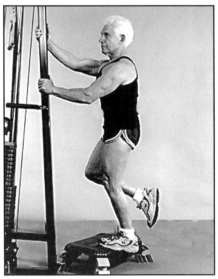

STANDING CALF RAISE ONE LEG
Same as above except using only one leg at a time. Most gyms have a Calf Machine where weight resistance can be applied on the shoulders.

CALVES

Start   Finish

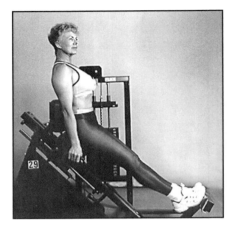 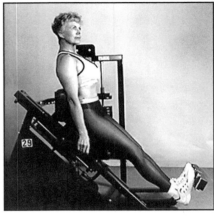

DONKEY CALF
The advantage of this machine is the weight is supported by your seat, reducing any strain on the back.

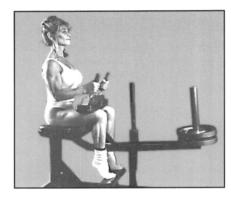 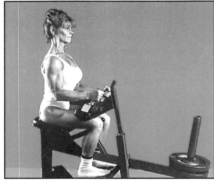

SEATED CALF
Push the heels down low, then raise on toes as high as possible for a maximum contraction.

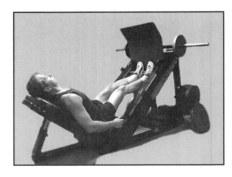 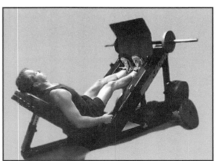

LEG PRESS CALF
Holding the up & down position for a two count will maximize results.

CHAPTER TWELVE

THE SHOULDERS
HELPFUL HINTS

The shoulders consist of the Deltoids and the Trapezius muscles. The Deltoids have three heads; the anterior, the posterior, and the medial. Whenever you push anything away from your body, you are using the anterior part of your Deltoid. All pressing movements employ this group of muscles.

All rowing movements use the posterior portion of the Deltoid. This group of muscles pulls things toward the body. With most people these muscles are more difficult to develop than the anterior deltoid, but greatly enhance the look of the shoulders when developed to the maximum.

The medial portion of the Deltoid is probably one of the most attractive muscle groups in the body. That's the area where the Biceps, Triceps and Deltoid all tie together. This also is the most difficult portion of the shoulders to develop. To work this area effectively, the arms must be moved laterally along side the body. The trick in isolating this group is to think of lifting the elbows rather than the hands. As you lift your elbows up from your sides, imagine you are holding a glass in each hand and you are slowly emptying water from this glass as you lift your elbows.

If done correctly, your elbows will rotate so that your baby finger is pointing to the ceiling. You should feel a slight burn in the middle of the Deltoid as you complete your set. Deltoid work demands the strictest form. If you are handling weights too heavy to do the exercise in strict form, I guarantee it is only a matter of time before elbow problems interrupt your training.

I cannot stress enough the use of strict form in all these deltoid movements. The Lats, Pecs, Biceps, Triceps and Trapezius all tie into the Deltoid, so this is a muscle that is easily damaged. I remember watching a Mr. America winner doing a Bent Over Lateral Raise on the crossover cables with just ten pounds. This man weighed over two hundred pounds and was using this tiny amount of weight, but he was doing the movement very slowly and with absolute precision. He had magnificent shoulders.

The Trapezius are muscles we use continually. One of the most powerful muscle groups in the body, they demand more stress for development than most other muscle areas. Whenever you lift anything from any position, you are using the Trapezius muscles.

The Shoulder Shrug is the most frequently used exercise for this group of muscles. When you are doing Shrugs, lift the shoulders in a straight line towards your ears. Do not rotate the shoulders, because this can lead to neck problems when heavy weights are employed. The Heavy Cleans and Upright Rowing motions are excellent for building up this muscle group. If you don't have wide shoulders, it's not a good idea to get the Trapezius too large as it will emphasize the narrowness of the shoulders. However, very few bodybuilders ever get their Deltoids too large. The bigger, thicker the Deltoids appear, the larger the shoulders will look. Nothing will make you look more like an advanced bodybuilder than wide Lats and thick Pecs, capped with large well rounded Delts

SHOULDERS
OVERHEAD PRESS

Start   *Finish*

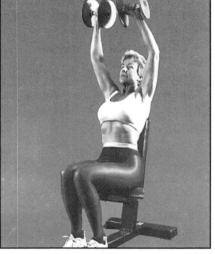

SEATED DMB OVERHEAD PRESS
Palms face forward throughout movement. Elbows parallel to shoulders in down position.

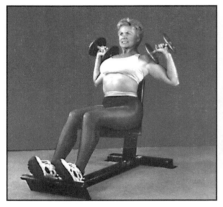

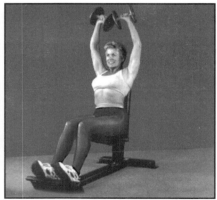

SEATED DMB "W" OVERHEAD PRESS
Elbows drop as low as possible in down position.

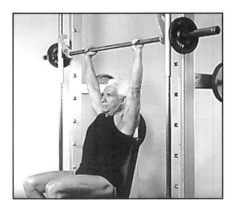

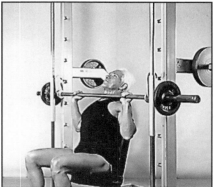

SMITH OVERHEAD PRESS
Keep the weight on the meaty part of the palm. This machine helps take the place of a "spotter""

SHOULDERS
OVERHEAD PRESS

Start

Finish

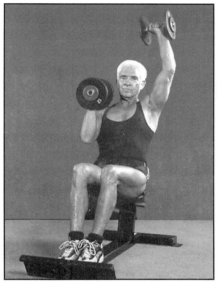
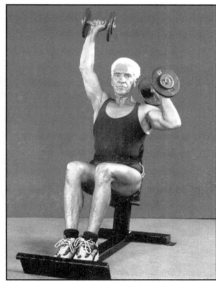

SEATED ALTERNATE OVERHEAD PRESS
Complete movement as shown.

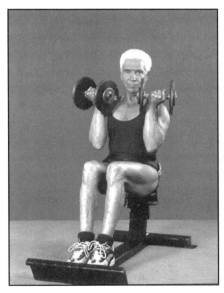
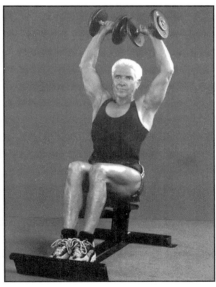

SEATED ARNOLD PRESS
Start with palms facing the shoulders. Rotate hands while pressing until palms face forward at the top.

SHOULDERS
STANDING

Start & Finish   *Middle*

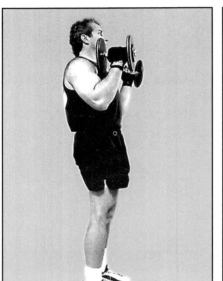 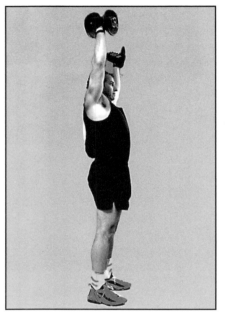

STANDING DMB OVERHEAD PRESS
Move the weight from shoulders to overhead in one movement.

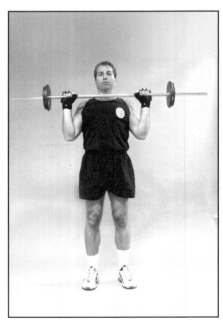 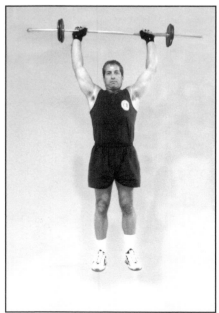

STANDING BBL OVERHEAD PRESS
Same as above.

SHOULDERS
UPRIGHT ROWS

Start   *Finish*

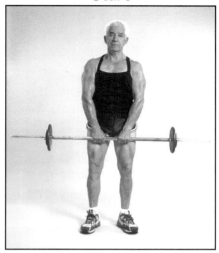 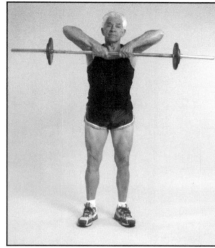

CLOSE GRIP
BBL UPRIGHT ROW
Raise elbows high to chin as shown. Keep BBL close to body.

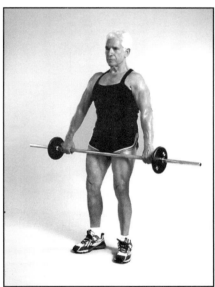 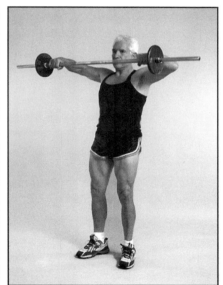

WIDE GRIP
BBL UPRIGHT ROW
Keep elbows high. Raise to nose level. Keep weight close to body while lifting bar.

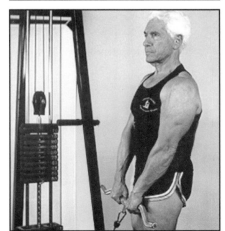 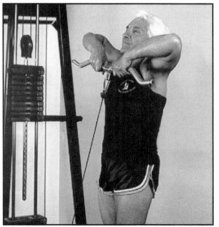

CABLE UPRIGHT ROW
Keep elbows high. Lift bar to chin level. Raise weight fast, lower it slowly.

SHOULDERS

Start *Finish*

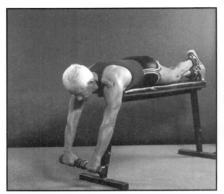 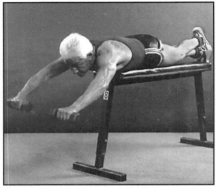

HIGH BENCH FRONT LATERALS
With straight arms try to raise weights as high as comfortably possible.

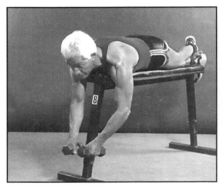 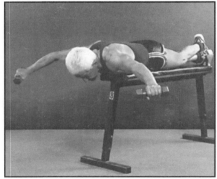

HIGH BENCH REAR LATERALS
Raise Dmbs with elbows high and slightly bent, keep hands forward.

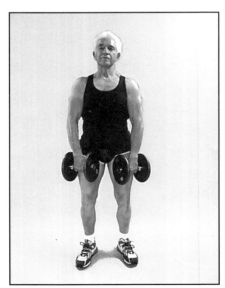 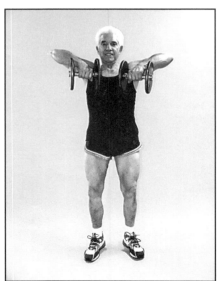

DMB UPRIGHT ROW
Same as above but with Dumbbells.

SHOULDERS
LATERAL RAISES

Start & Finish   Middle

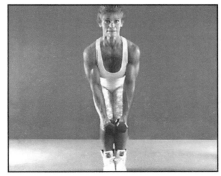 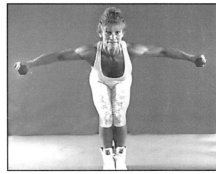

DMB BENT OVER LATERAL RAISES
Bent over, hold Dmbs with palms facing each other. Raise weight to sides with slight bend in elbows. Keep arms slightly forward of shoulder during movement.

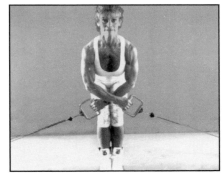 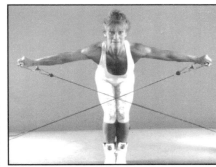

X-OVER BENT OVER LATERAL RAISES
Similar to above except using the cables.

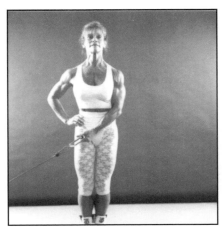 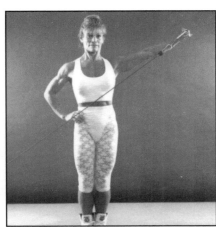

CABLE 1-ARM LATERAL RAISES
Same as above except standing upright using one arm at a time.

SHOULDERS
INCLINE BENCH LATERALS

Start   *Finish*

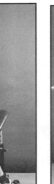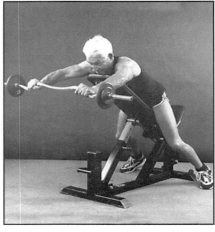

INCLINE BENCH BBL FRONT LATERALS
Lift weight in a straight motion to the front.

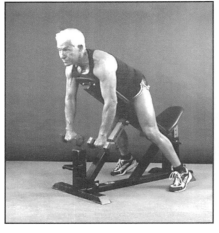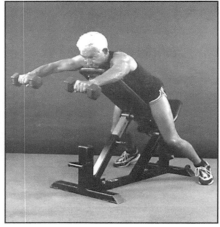

INCLINE BENCH DMB FRONT LATERALS
Same as above except with Dumbbells.

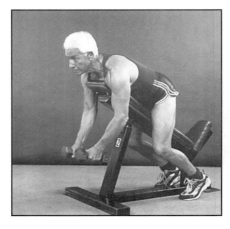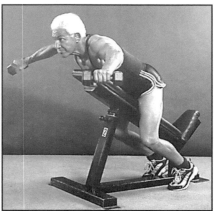

INCLINE BENCH REAR LATERALS
Raise Dmbs to the sides. With elbows high and slightly bent, keep hands forward of shoulders.

SHOULDERS
LATERAL RAISES

Start   Finish

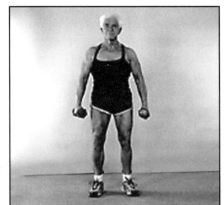 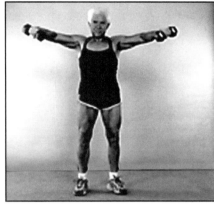

DMB SIDE LATERALS
With arms slightly bent, lift elbows laterally until they are just above shoulder height.

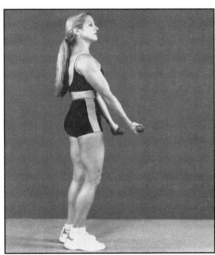 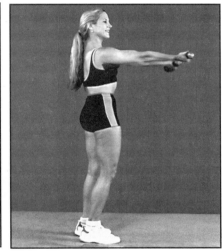

DMB FRONT LATERALS REVERSE GRIP
Hands in underhand position shoulder width apart. Lift Dmbs slightly higher than shoulder level.

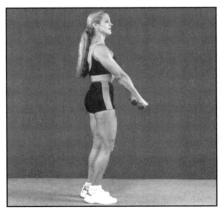 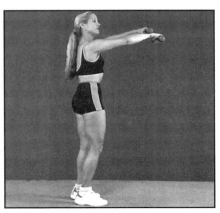

DMB FRONT LATERALS REGULAR GRIP
Same as above except hands in overhand position

SHOULDERS
LATERAL RAISES

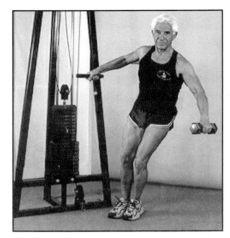 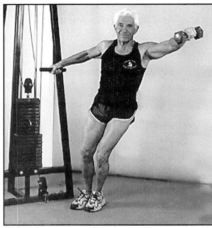

LEANING 1-ARM SIDE LATERALS
Think of lifting the elbow not the hand.

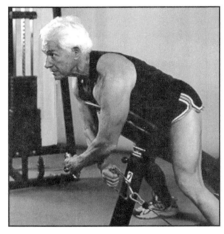 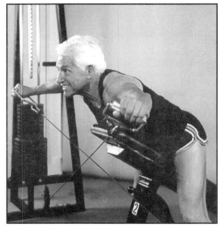

CABLE INCLINE REAR LATERALS
Hands should move forward as you raise them to the top position.

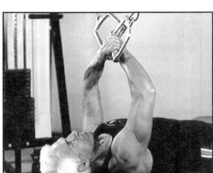 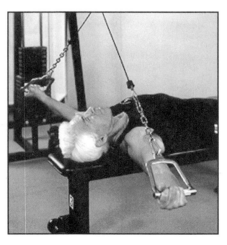

CABLE LYING REAR LATERALS
In all lateral exercises stop before your hands get to a resting position.

CHAPTER THIRTEEN

THE ARMS
HELPFUL HINTS

The upper arms consist of the Biceps (the front of the arm), the Triceps (the back of the arm) and the Brachialis (the part between the two). The function of the Biceps is to bend the arm forward. The Triceps straightens the arm. The Brachialis assists in bending the elbow.

The shape of the arm depends on your genetic background. Some arms will be high peaked while others will have a fuller, rounded appearance. No matter what your potential may be, lifting weights properly will give you pretty impressive arms. When looking at the human body, I don't think anything impresses people more than a big set of arms--where the Biceps are full and round and the Triceps have a deep "V" shaped groove running from the elbow to the Deltoid.

If the elbow is in good condition, all Biceps curling movements start with the weight hanging down to it's lowest position, (with a barbell, the bar against the thighs), and the elbows *almost* locked. The weight is then lifted, (with as little body move-ment as possible), to shoulder level. All Triceps Push-Downs positions should start at the level of the sternum, and with the elbows firmly held against your sides, push the bar down until the elbows are *lightly* locked at the bottom, with the handle touching your thighs.

Problem elbows are a different story. When rest and therapy have been tried, and there is still some irritation, you have at least two options. First, you can stop all Biceps work. Back work will keep the Biceps from losing too much size or strength. The back is strong enough to take pressure off the elbow and the secondary muscle in all back work is the Biceps so they will be exercised enough to keep them in pretty good shape.

The second choice is to limit the range of motion in your Biceps work. Experiment a little to find out where the problem presents itself. Many times just not extending the arm to it's fullest extension is enough to solve the problem. Simply do not lock out your arms at the lowest part of the exercise. Often just switching from a regular Curl to a Hammer Curl will take care of the problem. A little research on your part may turn up a form of Curl that causes no elbow irritation at all.

The same advice holds true for the Triceps when it comes to elbow problems. Age does take it's toll on our joints. While I am cautious in my training now that I am approaching the seventy-year mark, I still have an occasional problem. One of my trouble spots is an elbow problem when I do Triceps work. No matter how much trouble I have in this area, I can always do the Cross-Over Cable Triceps Kickback. This is a great Triceps exercise, and I will do it until the elbow has improved enough to add other Triceps movements to my routine. When I resume these exercises, I am very cautious to go slow and easy until I feel the muscle has recovered enough to fully train that area again.

I have always found there is some exercise I can do for an injured muscle group if I am persistent and willing to try new things. Remember muscles atrophy in seventy - two hours. No one wants to lose the gains they have made through hard work. I've seen what people look like that give up, and I don't want to go down that road. If you are this far in the Manual, I don't think you do either.

Forearms are one of the tough muscle groups to improve. Most people will get enough work on this area from just lifting the weights. You will find a hard back work out will leave your forearms really "pumped." All forms of the Curl will have some effect on the Forearms. If you wish to strengthen these muscles, you will find some great exercises in this book. Because this is a muscle we use constantly, the forearm takes more intensity than some of the other areas we work on.

For Forearms and Calves (another tough muscle group) we use high repetitions. If you are to have any type of success in this area, you really must be merciless in your training. High repetitions and little rest will get the best results when it comes to forearm improvement.

TRICEPS
FRENCH PRESS

Start & Finish   Middle

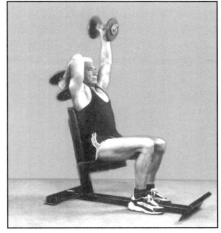 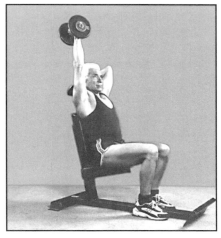

SEATED ALTERNATE DMB FRENCH PRESS

Keep elbows close to head.

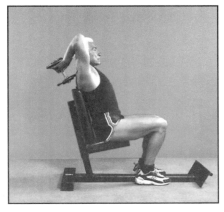 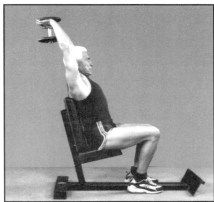

SEATED DMB FRENCH PRESS

Elbows should not move during exercise.

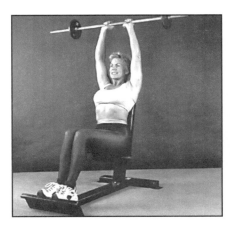 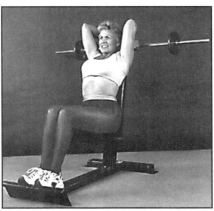

SEATED BBL FRENCH PRESS

Keep hands close together.

TRICEPS
KICKBACKS

Start & Finish   *Middle*

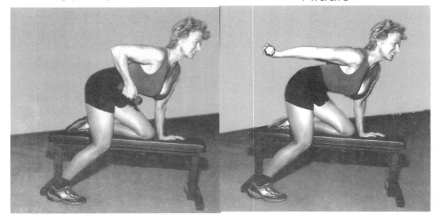

DMB KICKBACK
Keep elbow tight against body. Push hand back until elbow is as straight as possible.

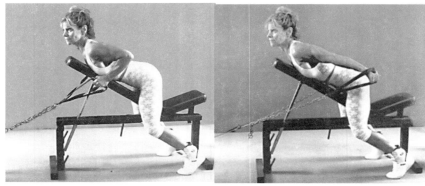

INCLINE CABLE KICKBACK
On Incline Bench

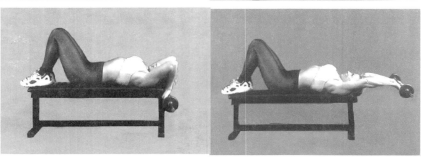

LYING BBL KICKBACKS
Keep upper arms at ear level.

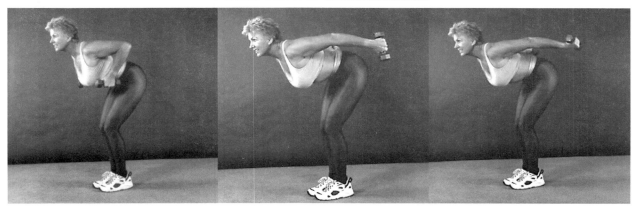

TRICEPS

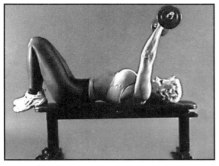 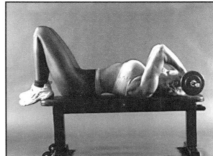

LYING BBL FRENCH PRESS
Try to keep elbows as stationary as possible in all French Press movements.

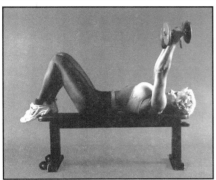 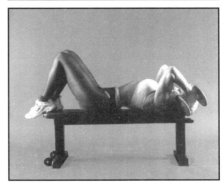

LYING DMB FRENCH PRESS
Keep elbows close to head.

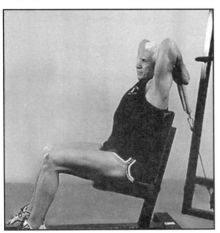 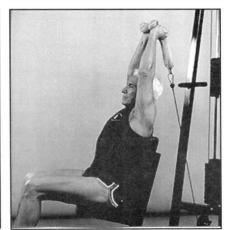

SEATED CABLE FRENCH PRESS
Let the hands come all the way down to the shoulders before starting upward movement.

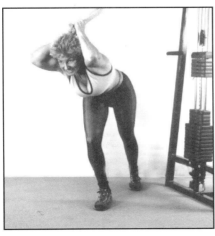 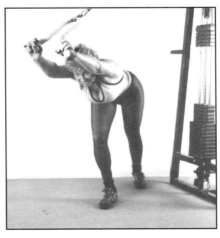

ROPE TRICEPS PUSH-AWAY
In the bent over position, hold one end of the rope in each hand. Bend the arms towards the shoulders as close as is comfortable. Push the rope away until your arms are fully extended, return to start position.

TRICEPS
PUSHDOWNS

Start & Finish   *Middle*

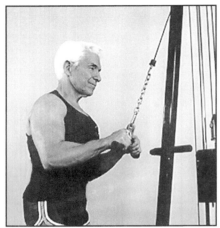 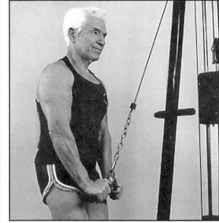

REGULAR TRICEPS PUSHDOWN
Be careful not to rock the body. Control the cable's upward movement for maximum results.

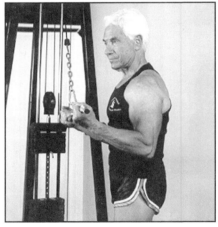 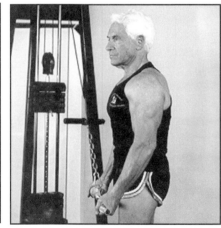

REVERSE GRIP PUSHDOWN
Maintain strict erect body position during exercise. Keep elbows tight against sides and do not move them once movement has started.

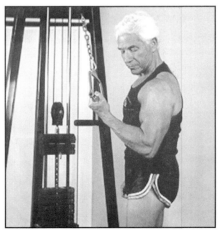 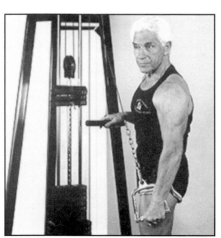

1-ARM PUSH-DOWN
Same as above. Note position of hands at start and finish of movement.

TRICEPS

Start & Finish   Middle

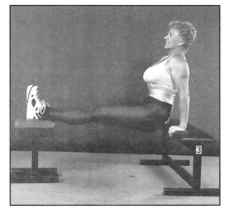 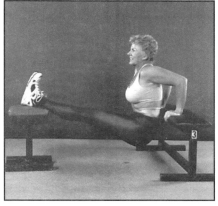

BENCH DIPS
The deeper you can allow your body to drop, the more you will feel the exercise in the Triceps.

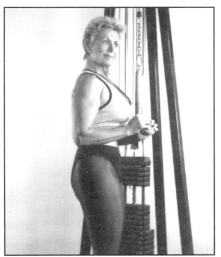 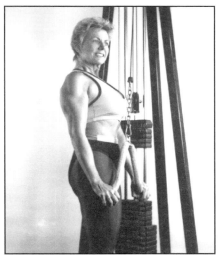

ROPE PUSH-DOWN
Start the exercise with hands together at chest height as illustrated. As you push down the rope, spread the hands so they are at the side of your thighs at the end of movement.

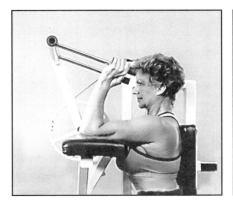 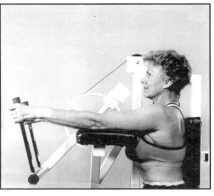

MACHINE PUSH-AWAY
Hold the arms of the machine as illustrated. Push the handles until your arms are straight, and return to starting position. Be sure to keep the elbows on the pad at all times.

TRICEPS
AND SHOULDERS COMBINATION

DMB FRENCH PRESS AND OVERHEAD PRESS COMBINATION

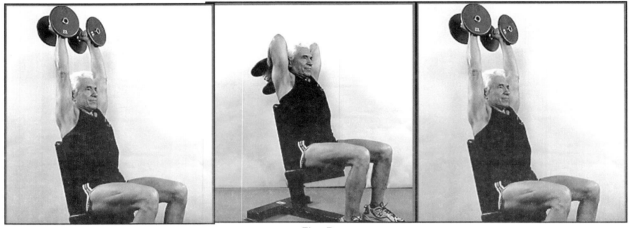

Fig. A   Fig. B   Fig. C

Palms face each other overhead. Lower weights keeping elbows close to head. Raise to start position.

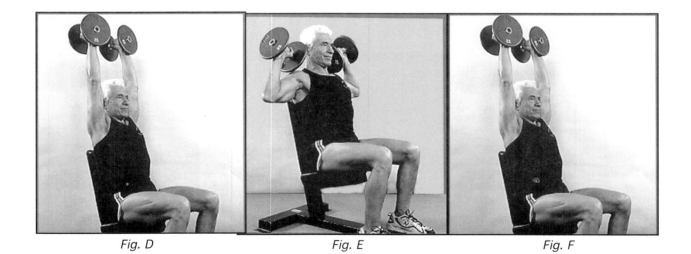

Fig. D   Fig. E   Fig. F

Palms twist to face forward while lowering weights to shoulders, and raise back overhead before twisting weights to face each other again as in *(Fig. A)*

BICEPS

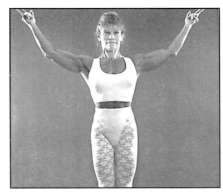 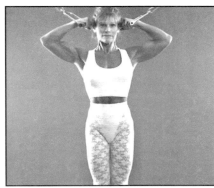

X-Over Cable Show Off Curls
For best results, keep elbows in line with shoulders.

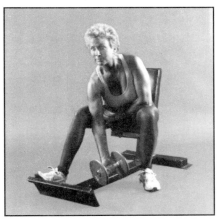 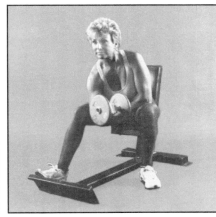

DMB Concentration Biceps Curls
Move hand slowly. Concentrate on the peak of the Biceps.

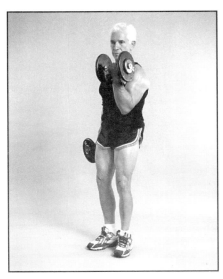 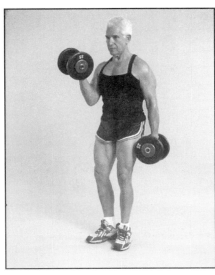

Alternate DMB Biceps Curls
Complete one arm at a time. Keep the body from swaying, let the Biceps do the work.

BICEPS
BLACK JACK CURLS

All pictures on this page are for this one exercise - done in three parts.

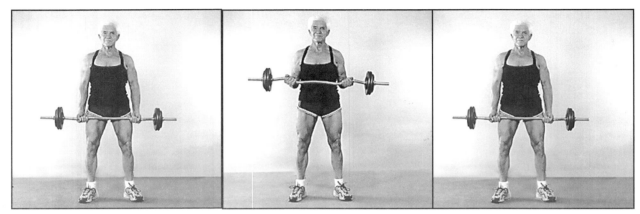

PART ONE: Arms fully extended then raised to half way up and lowered again. Do this lower part seven times.

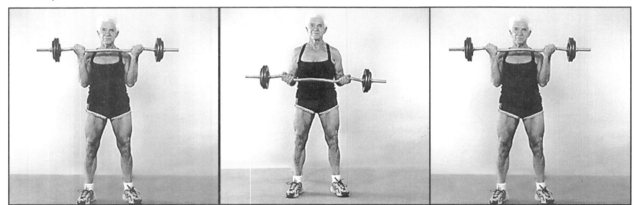

PART TWO: Arms come all the way up and then only half way down and up again. Do this upper part seven times.

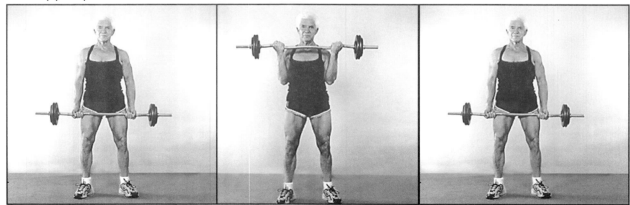

PART THREE: Seven full repetitions. The final part is the complete exercise. The Biceps should be really tired by this point.

7+7+7=21 BLACKJACK!

BICEPS
DUMBBELL CURLS

Start & Finish	Middle

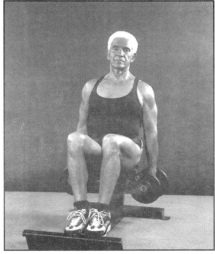 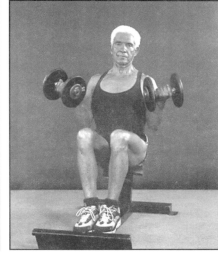

SEATED DMB CURLS
Palms twist up supinating the hands.

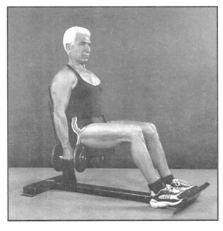 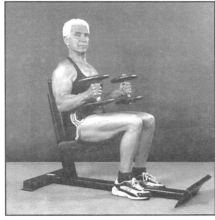

SEATED HAMMER CURLS
Palms stay in neutral position. Do not supinate.

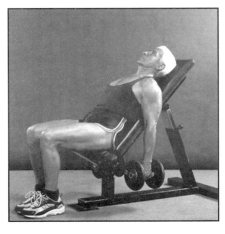 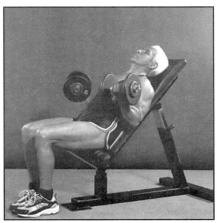

INCLINE DMB CURLS
Head and shoulders must stay on bench. Palms supinate as weights are raised.

BICEPS
STANDING BBL CURLS

Start & Finish

Middle

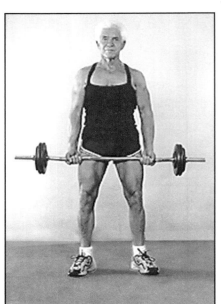 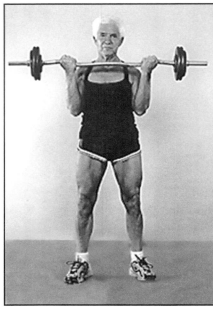

STANDING BBL CURLS
Lift the bar to your shoulders, without swinging the weight into position. Keep the elbows pressed against your ribs as you raise and lower the weight.

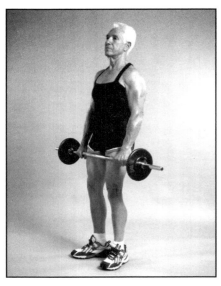 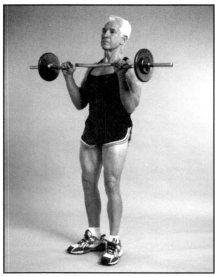

REVERSE GRIP BBL CURLS
Same as above except with overhand grip.

BICEPS
CABLES CURLS

Start & Finish   *Middle*

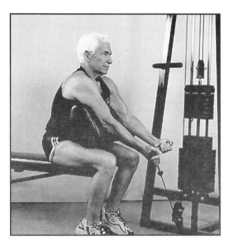
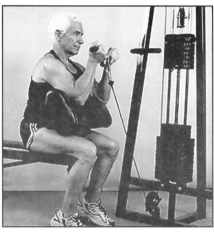

PREACHER CABLE CURLS
Keep pressure constant in cable curls so that you receive benefits from the negative part of the movement.

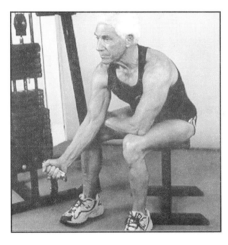
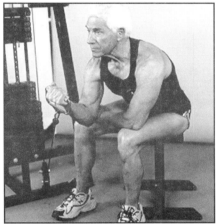

CABLE CONCENTRATION CURLS
As you curl weight up, aim the baby finger at the Deltoid. Bring weight to same shoulder as hand, not opposite.

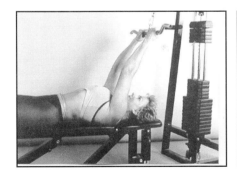
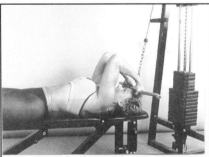

CABLE LYING BICEPS CURLS
Arms extended over forehead. Lower bar as shown. Return to starting position without moving the elbow.

BICEPS

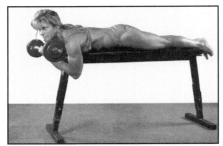 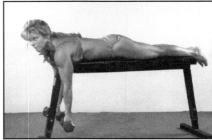

HIGH BENCH BBL CURLS
Keep elbows perpendicular to shoulders. Try to touch weight to forehead.

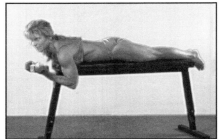 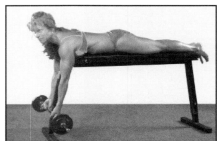

HIGH BENCH DMB CURLS
Same as above.

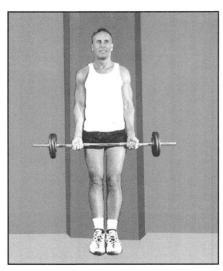 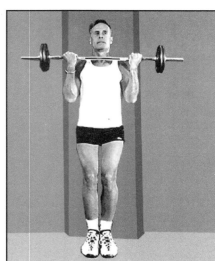

BBL WALL CURLS
Stand with feet about 12" from wall, knees bent slightly. Lean shoulders, head, and buttocks against wall for very strict curls.

BICEPS
CURLS ON BENCH

Start & Finish   Middle

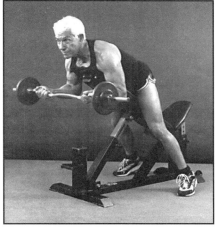

HANGING INCLINE BBL BICEPS CURLS
Keep elbows forward. Curl bar towards forehead.

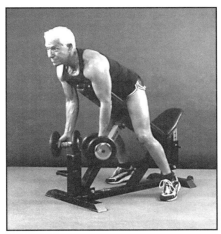 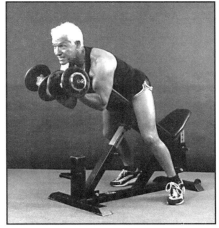

HANGING INCLINE DMB BICEPS CURLS
Same as above.

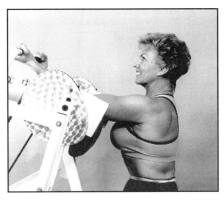 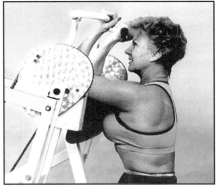

MACHINE BICEPS CURLS
Grasp the handles palm up and pull the weight towards your ears, then return to beginning. Keep the shoulders down, and elbows on pad at all times. Do not rock your body to help move the weight.

BICEPS
PREACHER CURLS

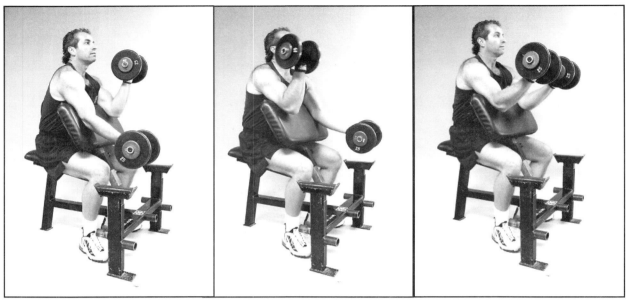

ALTERNATE PREACHER DMB CURLS
(shown above)

PREACHER DMB CURLS
(shown in top positon)

Keep elbows pressed against the pad through entire movement for maximum results. To protect elbows, do not straighten out the arms at the bottom of the exercise.

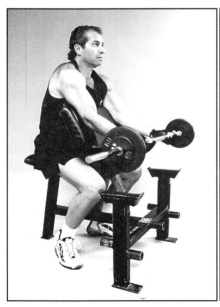 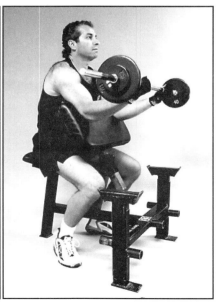

PREACHER BBL CURLS

CHAPTER FOURTEEN

THE NECK AND FOREARMS
HELPFUL HINTS

You will notice as you go through the workouts there are no exercises for the neck and forearms. The neck responds easily to exercises, and in my experiences here at our studio few people want larger necks. The neck is exercised just going through a regular routine. The forearms are constantly being used in all the upper body exercises. After a strenuous set of Curls or Pull-Downs your forearms will usually feel pretty pumped up.

For those of you who wish to exercise these body parts, I have included some movements in the illustrated part of this manual, and you can add these to your program if you so desire.

The neck is delicate so proceed slowly with any new exercises for this area. A sore neck is extremely uncomfortable. A few times in my career as a bodybuilder I attacked this part with too much enthusiasm and wound up with a neck so sore and stiff I could not move my head in any direction.

The forearms are worked continuously. Every time you clench your fist, pick something up with your hands, shake someone's hand, you are working your forearms. When we are working with clients, we are always telling them to relax their grip. Squeezing the handles of the weights tires out the forearm before you can feel the burn in the muscle you are trying to work.

Since this is a very difficult muscle to develop for most people, we urge you to use high repetitions when you are doing Forearm exercises. Because the forearm is such a tough muscle to work, at our Studio we recommend a minimum of twenty repetitions for this stubborn area. I would also encourage you to put all Forearm exercises at the end of the routine. It is difficult to work your biceps or back muscles if your forearms are exhausted.

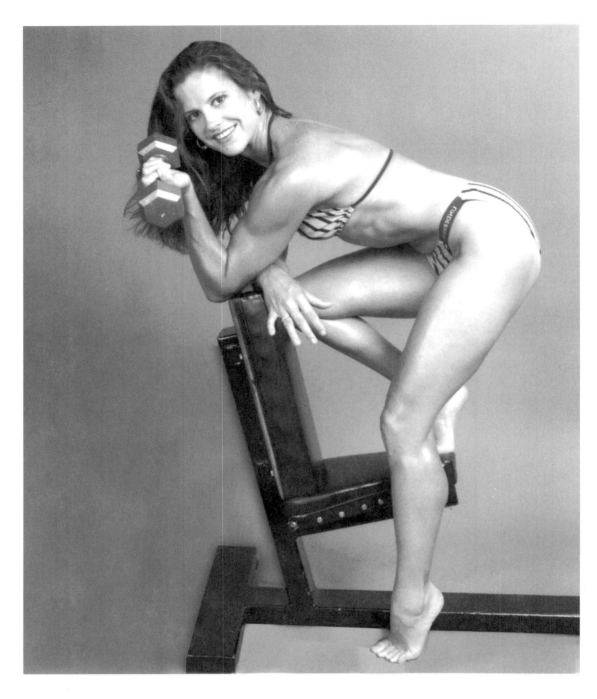

Our hard working editor, the ebullient Jeanie Cunningham.
Thank You

Index

FOREVER YOUNG

YOUR PERSONAL TRAINER

THE WORKOUT CHARTS

CHAPTER FIFTEEN

THE WORKOUT CHARTS
HOW TO USE THEM

The remainder of this manual deals with the Workout Charts themselves. The charts start with the easiest of the circuit training programs and progresses to workouts that are for the most advanced bodybuilders.

Copy the charts and keep a daily record of your progress. Mark down the dates, and the year, because it is always interesting to look back at your past performances. Like the food journal I mentioned in a previous chapter, people who keep records make more progress.

At the far left column of the chart you will see some numbers. Those numbers represent the equipment you need to perform that exercise. Simply refer to the numbers in the illustrations of the exercises, and you will see the equipment you need to use for a particular movement. If there is no number in the column, it means you are to use either a barbell or dumbbell in the standing position.

At the beginning of each group of charts, is an explanation of how these exercises work. For example, "Circuit

Training" is performed quite differently than the "6-20" Program. Read the description before you try the workout and you will get maximum results from your efforts.

Change your program at least once a month. The body adapts quickly! Every time you change your routine you use different muscle fibers. The more fibers you engage in your workouts, the more complete your total development. Changing your workouts will make them more interesting for you, and help you avoid boredom.

A partner can make a difference in your training. When you progress to using heavy poundages, you will need someone to spot you. Most importantly, a partner can keep a competitive edge in your workouts as well as keeping exercise a fun activity. Remember to keep records of your progress! Set realistic goals. Write those goals on your exercise charts. Follow these rules and you will be well on your way to reaching the goals you have set for yourself!

SAMPLE FILLED IN CHART

Fill in the weight under the WT and the repetitions in the blank column next to it.

EXERCISE	WT	
DMB Clean & Press	5	20
BBL Incline Press	40	15

If you see a bracket connecting two or more exercises, you are to complete all indicated without a rest break until you complete the group.

Leg Press	100	20
Leg Extension	30	20
Leg Curl	40	15

If there is a diagonal line through the square, it means you write the weight/repetitions in the same square. This leaves enough space to record multiple sets.

EXERCISE	WT	
Machine Donkey Calf	100 / 20	100 / 20

If you see the bracket and diagonal lines, then you complete the group, rest and repeat it again the second time.

Close Grip Pulldown	60 / 12
Seated Row	75 / 12

MEASUREMENTS CHART

Name: _____

Date:										
Weight										
Shoulders										
Chest										
Ribs										
Waist										
Hips fullest spot										
Left Thigh										
Right Thigh										
Knees										
Calves										
Rt. Arm Flexed										
Left Arm Flexed										

CHAPTER SIXTEEN

CIRCUIT TRAINING

Most people when they first get interested in training with weights see the "big guys" doing set after set of the same exercise. You will often see some enthusiastic advanced bodybuilder do eight to ten sets of one exercise for his chest or six to eight sets of one biceps exercise to get those body parts gigantic a little faster.

When a neophyte trainee tries to do the same thing as the advanced bodybuilder, the beginner usually gets such sore muscles that they can't move for days because of the pain caused by the excessive work they forced on muscles not yet prepared for this onslaught of fatiguing work.

CIRCUIT TRAINING is a way of preventing this pain and possible muscle damage from occurring. This type of training does only one exercise per body part then goes to another body part while the exercised muscle has time to recover. So you might do a Bench Press with a barbell to work your chest for your first exercise, then do a Pull down to the chin to work your back for your second, and later a Leg Press to exercise your thighs for your third. Later in the workout you might come back to the chest but this time you might use cable crossover Flys.

The advantage of **CIRCUIT TRAINING** is no muscle is overly stressed. If no rest is taken between exercises your stamina will increase, and the faster workout will burn more calories. At the beginning of your training, if the repetitions are kept high it will help toughen ligaments and tendons. This will help prevent injuries later when heavier training begins.

No matter what kind of program you are on, you must always keep trying to handle heavier weights. Muscles will only respond when they are stressed. That's why the weights are adjustable. Therefore, when you hit your goal, whether it be ten repetitions or twenty you must increase the weight. With the increase in poundage you should not be able to hit your target number. Stay with that weight until you hit that goal number then increase your weight again.

If you really want to increase your stamina and get as much weight loss benefits as possible, time your workouts and then try to cut your time down with each session. On programs one through six most beginners need forty-five minutes to an hour to complete the routine.

CIRCUIT TRAINING (Continued)

See whether you can work up to do the entire program twice in one hour! If you can do that much work that fast you are indeed in excellent cardiovascular condition and you will already see an improvement in your appearance.

Don't cheat yourself! Always use correct form, do not sacrifice form for speed or strength. Injuries are almost always a result of sloppy form in the exercise.

In this section of the manual you will see several workout sheets entitled Advanced Circuit Training. These programs were not designed for speed.

ADVANCED CIRCUIT TRAINING was developed as a break from the more difficult heavy training programs to give the joints a chance to recover from the stress of handling heavy weights for a month or two. If your body is not recovering from the training sessions, if there is any kind of pain in the elbows, knees, hips or back, if you're having trouble sleeping, eating, or lose interest in sex, it's time to back off on the heavy work and a perfect time to try Advanced Circuit Training. You must still try to increase

your poundages but there is more warm up time allowed on these programs and much more recovery time is allowed on each body part.

You will be pleasantly surprised at how much stronger you get on this routine though you may lose a little of the tone you had on the more difficult sessions. Don't worry, when you return to the more intense workouts you will be fresher and more enthusiastic about sculpturing your body. A month on this program should be enough to accomplish your purpose.

Name: _____   **Routine: Circuit Training #1**   **Date:** _____

EXERCISE	WT	WT	WT	WT	WT	WT	WT	WT	WT	WT	WT	WT	WT	WT	WT
Ab Routine #1															
Seated Alternate Dmb Overhead Press															
Wide Pulldown in Back															
BBL Flat Bench Press															
BBL Biceps Curl-standing															
Regular Triceps Pushdown															
Leg Extension															
Seated Leg Curl															
Pec Deck															
Dmb Shrugs															
Triceps Machine Pushaway															
BBL Upright Row-standing															
Leg Press															
Leg Press Calf															
Dmb Side Lateral Raises															
Seated Rowing Machine															
Seated Calf															
Sled Squat															

EXERCISE	WT	WT	WT	WT	WT	WT	WT	WT	WT	WT	WT	WT	WT	WT	WT	WT	WT	WT	WT	WT
Ab Routine #2																				
Hyperextensions																				
Dmb Swing																				
Lunge																				
Seated Dmb Overhead Press																				
Lying Leg Curl																				
Leg Extension																				
Dmb Flat Bench Press																				
Wide Grip Pulldown to Chin																				
Side Leg Machine in/out																				
Seated Calf																				
Dmb Incline Flys																				
Cable 1-arm Hi Pulldown																				
Leg Press																				
Calf on Leg Press																				
Seated Dmb French Press																				
Machine Biceps Curls																				
Sled Squat																				
Dmb Kickbacks																				
Seated Dmb Biceps Curls																				

EXERCISE	WT	WT	WT	WT	WT	WT	WT	WT	WT	WT	WT	WT	WT	WT	WT	WT
ABS #1 & #2 (Alternate)																
Hyperextensions																
Bent Knee Dmb Dead Lift																
Close Grip Pulldown																
Arnold Overhead Press																
BBL Lying French Press																
Black Jack BBL Biceps Curl																
Lunge																
Machine Donkey Calf																
Machine Incline Bench Press																
Seated Row																
Seated Calf																
Hack Squat																
BBL Preacher Biceps Curl																
Rope Triceps Pushdown																
Sled Squat																
X-over Cable Flat Flys																
Side Leg Machine in/out																
Dmb Side Lateral Raises																

Name: _____   **Routine: CIRCUIT TRAIN #4**   **Date:** _____

EXERCISE	WT	WT	WT	WT	WT	WT	WT	WT	WT	WT	WT	WT	WT	WT	WT	WT
ABS #3																
Dmb Clean & Press																
Dmb Incline Flys																
Machine Donkey Calf																
Round Grip Pulldown																
Good Mornings																
Dmb Flat Bench Press																
BBL Biceps Curls																
Machine Seated Overhead Press																
Leg Press																
Cable 1-arm Hi Pulldown																
Cable Upright Rows																
Machine Biceps Curls																
Seated Dmb French Press																
Sled Squat																
Dmb Shoulder Shrugs																
Machine Incline Press																
Seated Dmb Biceps Curls																
Regular Triceps Pushdown																
Side Leg Machine in/out																
Dmb Kickbacks																

Name: _____ **Routine: CIRCUIT TRAIN #5** **Date:** _____

EXERCISE	WT	WT	WT	WT	WT	WT	WT	WT	WT	WT	WT	WT	WT	WT	WT	WT
ABS																
GOOD MORNINGS																
Pec Deck																
Seated Leg Curl																
Smith Bench Press																
Cable Incline Low 1-Arm Pull																
Cable Lying Biceps Curls																
Seated Dmb Overhead Press																
X-Over Show-Off Curls																
Machine Pushaway																
Wide Grip Pulldown in Front																
Dmb Flat Flys																
Flat Bench																
BBL Triceps Kickbacks																
Leg Press High Plate																
Calf on Leg Press																
Dmb Leaning Side Laterals																
Sled Squat																
Seated Calf																
High Bench																
Dmb Rear Laterals																

EXERCISE	WT	WT	WT	WT	WT	WT	WT	WT	WT	WT	WT	WT	WT	WT	WT
ABS															
Hyperextensions															
BBL Hi Pulls (warm up)															
Machine Incline Bench Press															
Lying Leg Curl															
Seated Row															
Leg Extensions															
X-over Incline Flys															
Machine Shoulder Shrugs															
Side Leg Machine in/out															
Round Grip Pulldown															
Seated Leg Curl															
Seated Dmb Biceps Curls															
Lying Dmb French Press															
Sled Squats															
Dmb Concentration Curls															
Regular Triceps Pushdown															
Leg Press															
Calf on Leg Press															
Seated Side Lateral Raises															
Dmb 1-arm Kickbacks															
Seated Calf															

Name: _____   **Routine:** ADVANCED CIRCUIT #1   **Date:** _____

EXERCISE	WT	WT	WT	WT	WT	WT	WT	WT	WT	WT	WT	WT	WT	WT	WT	WT	WT
ABS																	
Hyperextensions																	
(warm up) Flat Bench Press																	
Seated Leg Curl																	
Dmb Flat Bench Press																	
Seated Calf																	
(warm up) Machine Incline Bench Press																	
Machine Shrugs																	
Machine Incline Bench Press																	
Cable 1-arm Hi Pulldown																	
Seated Dmb Overhead Press																	
Machine Triceps Pushaway																	
BBL Preacher Biceps Curl																	
X-over Incline Flys																	
Wide Grip Pulldown to Chin																	
(warm up) Leg Press																	
Leg Press																	
Dmb Leaning Side Laterals																	
Sled Squat																	
Machine Donkey Calf																	
Dmb Incline Biceps Curls																	
X-over Lying Rear Laterals																	

111

EXERCISE	WT	WT	WT	WT	WT	WT	WT	WT	WT	WT	WT	WT	WT	WT
Abs & Hyperextensions														
(warm up) Dmb Bent Arm Pullover & Press														
BBL Cleans (warm up)														
Bent Arm Pullover & Press														
BBL Power Cleans														
Incline Bench BBL Front Lateral Raise														
Leg Extension														
X-over Standing Fly														
BBL Bent Leg Dead Lift														
High Bench Dmb Rear Laterals														
Leg Curl														
Hanging Incline BBL Curls														
Lying BBL Kickbacks														
Cable Lying Biceps Curls														
Machine Donkey Calves														
High Bench Rows BBL Reverse Grip														
Dmb Fly & Press Combo														
Leg Press														
Cable 1-Arm Lateral Raise														
Dmb Seated French Press & Overhead Press Combo														

EXERCISE	WT	WT	WT	WT	WT	WT	WT	WT	WT	WT	WT	WT	WT	WT
Abs & Hyperextensions														
(warm up) Machine Incline Bench Press														
Straight Arm Pullover														
(warm up) Close Grip Pulldown														
Machine Incline Bench Press														
Dmb Shoulder Shrugs														
Close Grip Pulldown														
Seated French Press														
Seated Calf														
Hack Squat (warm up)														
BBL Biceps Curls														
Hack Squat														
Bent Arm Pullover														
Arnold Overhead Press														
Bent Over Dmb Kickbacks														
Side Lateral Raises														
Seated Dmb Biceps Curls														
Upright Rows														
Leg Press (warm up)														
Leg Press Calf														
Leg Press														
Cable Incline Low 1-arm Pull														

Name: _____   **Routine: ADVANCED #4 HIGH INTENSITY (As little Rest as Possible) Date:** _____

EXERCISE	WT	WT	WT	WT	WT	WT	WT	WT	WT	WT	WT	WT	WT	WT	WT	WT	WT	WT
Abs & Hyperextensions																		
Clean & Press																		
Sled Squat																		
Straight Arm Pullover																		
Machine Incline Bench Press																		
Leg Press																		
Straight Arm Pullover																		
Close Grip Pulldown																		
Machine Triceps Pushaway																		
Hack Squat																		
Bent Arm Pullover																		
Dmb Shoulder Shrug																		
BBL Preacher Curl																		
Seated French Press																		
Dmb Flat Bench Press																		
Incline Bench Rear Laterals																		
High Bench Rear Laterals																		
Incline Bench Front Laterals																		
Standing Side Laterals																		
Seated Leg Curl																		
Seated Calf																		
Machine Donkey Calf																		

EXERCISE	WT	WT	WT	WT	WT	WT	WT	WT	WT	WT	WT	WT	WT	WT	WT	WT	WT
ABS																	
warm up Machine Incline Bench Press																	
Leg Extension - warm up																	
Machine Incline Bench Press																	
Leg Extension																	
Leg Press - warm up																	
Seated Calf																	
Leg Press - High Plate																	
Dmb Flat Bench Fly																	
Seated Rowing Machine																	
Sled Squat - warm up																	
Tricep Pushdown																	
Sled Squat																	
Staight Arm Pullover																	
Wide Grip Pulldown																	
X-Over Lying Rear Laterals																	
Seated Dmb Hammer Curls																	
Hack Squat																	
Dmb Bent Arm Pullover																	
Cable Lying Bicep Curls																	
Incline Cable Kickbacks																	
Leg Press - Low plate																	

CHAPTER SEVENTEEN

PUSH PULL

PUSH PULL programs usually follow the **CIRCUIT TRAINING** programs. It is more intensive than Circuit Training but not as intense as the **TOTAL BODY** programs. Basically, the trainee works opposing muscles in double sets. For example, the person working out might do an exercise for the chest, which he would follow immediately with a back exercise.

The idea is, that when a person is doing a Chest exercise, like a Bench Press, he is doing a pushing movement. When he does a Back exercise, like a "rowing" motion, he is doing a pulling movement. So when the Chest is working, the Back is resting. Since one is pushing and one is pulling, there is no need to rest between "Push-Pull" sets.

In this program, Chest is combined with Back, Biceps combined with Triceps, Anterior Deltoid coupled with Posterior Deltoid (shoulders), Quadriceps of the thighs worked with the Hamstrings and "Glutes" etc.

The trick here is not to rest between combinations. Again, if you do an Incline Bench Fly followed by a Wide Grip Lat Pulldown, do not rest between exercises. The rest pause comes after the second movement. It's the same with all the body parts. A seated dumbbell Biceps Curl followed by a Triceps Pushdown needs no rest. Resting after the Triceps Pushdown is O.K.

Remember, when you hit the goal set for the number of repetitions you wish to reach, increase the weight. The body must constantly be challenged for there to be any improvement. If there is no stress, there is no gain!

Name: _____   **Routine:** _____   **PUSH - PULL #1**   **Date:** _____

EXERCISE	WT	WT	WT	WT	WT	WT	WT	WT	WT	WT	WT	WT	WT	WT	WT	WT
ABS																
Hyperextensions																
BBL Hi-Pulls (warm up)																
Machine Incline Press																
Wide Pulldown in Front																
Flat Dmb Bench Press																
Seated Row Machine																
Sled Squat																
Lying Leg Curl																
Hack Squat																
Seated Leg Curl																
Arnold Dmb Overhead Press																
Machine Shoulder Shrugs																
Dmb Side Lateral Raises																
Dmb 1-arm Kickbacks																
Standing BBL Biceps Curl																
Seated Dmb French Press																
Machine Biceps Curl																
Rope Triceps Pushdown																
Seated Dmb Biceps Curl																
Machine Donkey Calf																

117

Name: _____ **Routine: PUSH - PULL #2** **Date:** _____

EXERCISE	WT	WT	WT	WT	WT	WT	WT	WT	WT	WT	WT	WT	WT	WT	WT	WT
ABS																
Hyperextensions																
Dmb Clean & Press																
Smith Flat Bench Press																
Close Grip Pulldown																
Incline Dmb Bench Press																
Cable Incline Low 1-Arm Pull																
BBL Upright Row																
Seated Dmb Overhead Press																
Leaning 1-arm Side Laterals																
(Sitting Optional) Dmb palms up Front Laterals																
Leg Extensions																
Seated Leg Curl																
Leg Press																
Hack Squat																
Lying Cable Biceps Curls																
Machine Triceps Pushaway																
Cable Preacher Curl																
Rope Triceps Pushdown																
Machine Shoulder Shrugs																
Seated Calf																

118

EXERCISE	WT	WT	WT	WT	WT	WT	WT	WT	WT	WT	WT	WT	WT	WT
ABS														
Good Mornings														
Clean & Press (warm up)														
Dmb Flat Bench Press														
Wide Pulldown in Back														
Dmb Incline Bench Press														
Wide Pulldown in Front														
Smith Decline Bench Press														
Close Grip Pulldown														
X-over Lying Rear Laterals														
Dmb Shoulder Shrugs														
Seated Dmb Overhead Press														
Seated Dmb Biceps Curl														
Regular Triceps Pushdown														
Standing BBL Curl														
Rope Triceps Pushdown														
Machine Biceps Curls														
Reverse Triceps Pushdown														
Leg Press (high plate)														
Sled Squat														
Leg Press (low plate)														
Calves on Leg Press														
Machine Donkey Calf														

Name: _____   Routine: _____   PUSH - PULL #4   Date: _____

EXERCISE	WT	WT	WT	WT	WT	WT	WT	WT	WT	WT	WT	WT	WT	WT	WT	WT
ABS																
Hyperextensions																
(warm up Chest & Back)																
Flat Flys																
Close Grip Pulldown																
Smith Decline Bench Press																
Seated Row																
Leg Extension																
Seated Leg Curl																
Flat Fly & Press Combo																
Reverse Grip Pulldown																
Machine Donkey Calf																
Machine Shoulder Shrugs																
High Bench Dmb Front Laterals																
Seated Dmb Overhead Press																
Incline Hanging BBL Biceps Curls																
Lying BBL Triceps Kickback																
Preacher BBL Biceps Curls																
Regular Triceps Pushdown																
Dmb Concentration Curls																
Incline Cable Triceps Kickbacks																
Hack Squat																
Leg Press																

Name: _____   Routine: _____   PUSH - PULL #5   Date: _____

EXERCISE	WT	WT	WT	WT	WT	WT	WT	WT	WT	WT	WT	WT	WT	WT	WT	WT
ABS																
Hyperextensions																
Leg Press (warm up)																
Close Grip Pulldown																
Dmb Incline Press																
Leg Extension																
Leg Press																
Wide Grip Pulldown in Front																
BBL Flat Bench Press																
Side Leg Machine In & Out																
Side Leg Machine to Back																
Lying Cable Biceps Curls																
Triceps Machine Pushaway																
Leg Curl																
Sled Squat																
Side Lateral Raises																
X-Over Lying Rear Laterals																
Leg Extensions																
Leg Curl																
Dmb Shoulder Shrugs																
BBL Biceps Curl																
BBL Upright Row																
Triceps Pushdown																

CHAPTER EIGHTEEN

TOTAL BODY

After you have been training for a few months, your body is now conditioned to do more arduous workouts. Keeping in mind the only way the body will continue to improve is to make the sessions with the weights more demanding every time you train. **TOTAL BODY** Programs are the next step.

In these sessions the exercises for each muscle group are closer together so there is now _less_ rest time for the muscle to recover than in previous workouts.

With **CIRCUIT TRAINING** Programs a muscle group such as the chest rested while you exercised your back or legs, giving these muscles plenty of rest time before you worked them again. **TOTAL BODY** Programs are designed to do from two to six exercises in a row per muscle before going to another muscle group. This is much more demanding than the past programs we have discussed.

The different programs in this section are to be followed in a specific manner for them to be effective. It is of the utmost importance that you try to go to failure on each set. That means you must push as hard as you can on each exercise until you positively cannot do one more repetition. This is quite demanding on your body but the results will astound you. If you do not see a noticeable change in three months, you are doing something wrong, re-read the text and make sure you are touching all the points!

You will find two programs in this section that deal specifically with **SHOULDER PROBLEMS.** The most common complaint in health clubs is the damaged Deltoids. Most of those problems come from handling too much weight with improper form. The exercises in these routines minimize the use of the Deltoids so that you can continue to work out, and still give your shoulders a chance to "cool off." The same principles apply to any area that has been slightly injured. Of course, if the area continues to deteriorate, consult a sports medicine doctor.

Name: _____   Routine: TOTAL BODY #1 (3 in a row)   Date: _____

EXERCISE	WT	WT	WT	WT	WT	WT	WT	WT	WT	WT	WT	WT	WT	WT	WT
Abs															
Dmb Clean & Press															
Close Grip Pulldown															
Dmb Bent Arm Pullover															
Dmb One Arm Row															
Dmb Flat Flys															
Flat BBL Bench Press															
Incline Dmb Bench Press															
Seated Calf															
Leg Press Calf															
BBL Upright Row															
Seated Dmb Overhead Press															
Dmb Side Lateral Raises															
Seated Dmb Biceps Curl															
BBL Biceps Curl															
Regular Triceps Pushdown															
Lying BBL French Press															
Machine Triceps Pushaway															
Hack Squat															
Leg Press															
Sled Squat															

Name: _____   Routine: **TOTAL BODY #2**   (3 in a row)   Date: _____

EXERCISE	WT	WT	WT	WT	WT	WT	WT	WT	WT	WT	WT	WT	WT	WT	WT	WT
ABS																
Hyperextensions																
Cable 1-arm Hi Pulldown																
Dmb One Arm Row																
Cable Incline Low 1-arm Pull																
BBL Bench Press																
Dmb Flat Bench Press																
Decline Smith Bench Press																
Dmb Seated Overhead Press																
Side Lateral Raises																
Leg Press Calf																
Cable Preacher Biceps Curl																
Seated Dmb Biceps Curls																
Preacher BBL Biceps Curl																
Seated French Press																
Cable Incline Kickbacks																
Rope Overhead Pushaway																
Leg Press																
Hack Squat																
Seated Calf																
Sled Squat																
Leg Curl																

124

EXERCISE	WT	WT	WT	WT	WT	WT	WT	WT	WT	WT	WT	WT	WT	WT	WT	WT
ABS & Hyperextensions																
X-over Incline Cable Flys																
Machine Incline Bench Press																
Dmb Flat (palms in) Press																
Dmb Incline (palms in) Press																
Round Grip Pulldown Shrugs																
Round Grip Pulldown to Chin																
Machine Seated Row																
Close Grip Pulldown to Chin																
X-over Lying Rear Laterals																
Dmb Side Lateral Raises																
X-over Incline Rear laterals																
Machine Biceps Curl																
Cable Preacher Biceps Curl																
BBL Standing Biceps Curl																
Regular Triceps Pushdown																
Machine Triceps Pushaway																
Dmb Seated French Press																
Leg Extensions																
Sled Squat																
Hack Squat																
Leg Press & Calf																

Routine: TOTAL BODY For Shoulder Problems #1 Date: _____

EXERCISE	WT	WT	WT	WT	WT	WT	WT	WT	WT	WT	WT	WT	WT	WT
ABS														
Leg Press (warm up)														
Leg Extension														
Leg Press														
(warm up) Close Grip Pulldown														
Tricep Pushdown														
Close Grip Pulldown														
Tricep Pushdown														
Close Grip Pulldown														
Machine Tricep Pushaway														
High Bench BBL Row														
Dmb Triceps Kickbacks														
Machine Donkey Calf														
Sled Squat														
Leg Curl														
Cable Preacher Curl														
Hack Squat														
BBL Preacher Curl														
Seated Calf														
Incline Rear Lateral Raises														
Machine Biceps Curls														
High Bench Rear Laterals														
(your choice) Dmb Incline or Flat Bench Press														

Name: _____   **Routine: TOTAL BODY For Shoulder Problems #2**   **Date:** _____

EXERCISE	WT	WT	WT	WT	WT	WT	WT	WT	WT	WT	WT	WT	WT	WT	WT	WT
ABS																
Hyperextensions																
Seated Row																
Regular Triceps Pushdown																
High Bench Dmb Row																
Triceps Machine Pushaway																
Leg Press																
Leg Press Calf																
BBL Reverse Grip High Bench Row																
Dmb Seated Biceps Curls																
Incline or Flat BBL Bench Press																
Machine Biceps Curls																
Sled Squat																
Seated Calf																
BBL Biceps Curls																
Rope Triceps Pushaway																
Hack Squat																
Machine Donkey Calf																
Wide Grip Pulldown																
Seated Row																
Leg Extension																
Seated Leg Curl																

ADVANCED TOTAL BODY

This section deals with a variety of programs more advanced than those done up to this point. Each routine works the entire body and is completed in one session. Keep in mind always that the body adapts easily. Any routine you do for more than a month is probably not going to be effective. To make your workouts productive and interesting, we offer a wide variety of workouts in this section.

MASS BUILDING: This routine is designed to increase muscle mass and strength. Years ago a magazine called *Strength and Health* constantly preached in its publication "Train for strength and shape will follow."

On this program you will notice with each body part you do fewer repetitions as you complete each set. That's because you must make each set heavier than the one before. On the ten, eight and four repetition sets, go to failure on each exercise. As soon as you can complete the given number of repetitions on each set, you must increase the weight. When you increase the poundage, strict form is still imperative. Sloppy form with heavy weights will only lead to injuries.

When you add additional plates to the bars, the repetitions and then immediately cut the poundage in half and do will go down. That's O.K.. Stay with that poundage until you make that predetermined goal. Whenever you achieve the number you are striving for in a set, you have to increase the weight while continuing to maintain good form. If you go three or four weeks without increasing your performance,

you are doing something wrong. Try to figure out your problem. The answer may be to get a training partner to make you push harder on each movement. Possibly you have to change some of the exercises. Whatever you try, if you are not getting results go off this program and try another routine. You can always come back to the Mass Building Program another time.

6-20 WORKOUT: Each muscle has two kinds of fibers, these are the *Fast Twitch* and *Slow Twitch Fibers*. *Fast twitch* fibers are used for explosive movements. Sprinters have many *fast twitch* muscles, while Marathon runners have more *Slow twitch* fibers.

To build the body, we lift heavy weights as fast as possible to employ the *fast twitch* fibers, while lighter weights with higher repetitions at a moderate rate use the *slow twitch* fibers. Since they are different fibers within the same muscle, no rest is needed when going from one fiber group to the other.

You must take a weight you can barely lift for six repetitions and then immediately cut the poundage in half and do twentyrepetitions with that weight. The poundage in the twenty repetition range will vary with that cutting in half, depending on how many *slow twitch* fibers you have. Experiment a little to find what percentage will work for you. It is important to keep in mind to go to failure on both the

ADVANCED TOTAL BODY

"6 and the 20" rep sets.

SUPER-SETS: If you have hit a sticking point, or if you are trying to get more definition in your muscles, Super-Sets would be the program to try. In this workout you do two sets in a row of different exercises for the same body part. For example, if you are working the chest you might do a set of Barbell Flat Bench Presses combined with a set of Incline Bench Flys. No rest is taken between these two sets, and you must go to failure on each exercise.

The two combined exercises are considered one Super-Set. In these programs there are several Super-Sets for each body part. If you are training for size, take a rest pause of one to three minutes between each of the Super-Sets. On the other hand, if definition is your goal, take as little rest as possible between these sets. This will seem very difficult because of the intensity of this type of training. With persistence, you can cut this interval to under thirty seconds.

How badly you want that definition will determine how fast you reach your goal!

DESCENDING SETS: Whenever you do a set of exercises, the only repetitions that count as far as the muscle growth is concerned are the last few reps. If you are doing a set of ten repetitions, the first eight reps are just to tire you

enough so that you get the full benefit from the last two. When you are doing Descending Sets, the first set should be ten repetitions. Then, immediately the weight is dropped enough so that only three or four reps can be achieved, and then again without pause a third set should be done attempting to get two or three reps.

Descending only works if you go to failure on each set. This is one of the toughest of the programs. If you are getting six or seven reps on the second set, you did not go to failure on the first or you lightened the weight too much. The same applies on the third set. If you are getting five or six reps on the third set, you are definitely doing something wrong. I would certainly follow this program with a circuit training workout to give the body a chance to rest for a while.

A good program to alternate with the more strenuous workouts in this section is the "3 In A Row" program referred to in the previous chapter. For example, you might try the "6-20" program for four weeks and then try the "3 In A Row" for two weeks. However, if you are really fatigued after a four-week stint, go back to "Circuit Training" for two weeks before resuming the harder sessions.

Remember, the body adapts to the exercises in about four weeks. To get results, change the programs regularly. The more the muscles are shocked the faster they gain size and strength.

EXERCISE	WT	WT	WT	WT	WT	WT	WT	WT	WT	WT	WT	WT	WT	WT	WT
ABS															
BBL Good Mornings															
Pec Deck															
Flat BBL Bench Press															
Seated Leg Curl															
Leg Machine – Back															
Seated Row Machine															
Round Grip Pulldown															
Seated Calf															
Sled Squat															
Leg Extension															
Leg Machine in/out															
Machine Overhead Press															
Lying Dmb French Press															
Triceps Rope Pushdown															
Leaning 1-arm Side Laterals															
Seated Dmb Biceps Curls															
Preacher BBL Biceps Curl															
Machine Shrugs															
Lying Leg Curl															
Leg Press															
Leg Press Calf															

Name: _____ **Routine: ADVANCED TOTAL #2 w/Super-Sets** **Date:** _____

EXERCISE	WT	WT	WT	WT	WT	WT	WT	WT	WT	WT	WT	WT	WT	WT	WT
AB Routine #3															
Hyperextensions															
⬚ Wide Pulldown in Front															
Cable 1-arm Pulldown															
Leg Machine in/out															
Leg Machine Back															
⬚ Incline Dmb Bench Press															
Pec Deck															
⬚ Lying Leg Curl															
Leg Extension															
Dmb Side Lateral Raises															
⬚ Seated Leg Curl															
Sled Squat															
⬚ Seated Dmb Overhead Press															
Dmb Upright Row															
Leg Press															
Leg Press Calf															
Seated Calf															
⬚ Cable Preacher Biceps Curl															
BBL Biceps Curl															
⬚ Alternate Dmb French Press															
Bent Over Dmb Kick Back															

Name: _____   **Routine: ADVANCED TOTAL #3 W/Super-Sets**   **Date:** _____

EXERCISE	WT	WT	WT	WT	WT	WT	WT	WT	WT	WT	WT	WT	WT	WT	WT
ABS															
Good Mornings															
BBL Clean & Press															
Flat Dmb Bench Press															
Incline Dmb Fly															
Stretch Chest															
Close Grip Pulldown															
Seated Row															
Stretch Back															
Leg Extension															
Sled Squat															
Lying Leg Curl															
Hack Squat															
Leg Press High Plate															
Stretch Legs															
Dmb Arnold Press															
Side Laterals															
Cable Incline Kickback															
Regular Pushdown															
BBL Biceps Curl															
Machine Biceps Curl															

132

Routine: ADVANCED TOTAL #4 w/Descending   Date: _____

EXERCISE	WT	WT	WT	WT	WT	WT	WT	WT	WT	WT	WT	WT	WT	WT
ABS #1, 2, 3 (Alternate)														
BBL Clean & Press														
Close Grip Pulldown														
Cable Standing Straight Arm Pushdown														
Cable 1-Arm High Pulldown (descending)														
Dmb Flat Flys														
BBL Close Grip Straight Arm Pullover														
Dmb Incline Flys (descending)														
Leg Extension														
Hack Squat														
Leg Press High (descending)														
X-over Bent Over Laterals														
Dmb Seated "W" Press (descending)														
Dmb Preacher Biceps Curl														
BBL Biceps Curl (descending)														
Rope Overhead Pushaway														
Regular Triceps Pushdown (descending)														
Machine Donkey Calves														

EXERCISE	WT	WT	WT	WT	WT	WT	WT	WT	WT	WT	WT	WT	WT	WT	WT	WT
ABS																
Dmb Clean & Press																
X-over Incline Flys																
Dmb Incline Bench Press																
Smith Flat Bench Press																
(descending)																
Seated Calf (3 positions)																
Close Grip Pulldown																
Seated Row (high handles)																
Wide Grip Pulldown to Chin																
(descending)																
Seated Leg Curl																
Leg Extension																
Leg Press																
(descend every other time)																
Sled Squat																
(descend every other time)																
Arnold Overhead Press																
Side Laterals																
Machine Biceps Curls																
Preacher Biceps Curls																
BBL Lying French Press																
Incline Cable Kickbacks																

EXERCISE	WT	WT	WT	WT	WT	WT	WT	WT	WT	WT	WT	WT	WT	WT	WT
ABS															
Hyperextensions															
warm up X-Over Flys															
X-Over Incline Flys															
Machine Incline Bench Press															
Dmb Flat Bench Press															
Wide Pulldown in Front															
Seated Row (low handles)															
Cable 1-Arm Hi Pulldown															
Seated Dmb "W" Overhead Press															
X-Over Lying Rear Laterals															
Wide Grip BBL Upright Row															
Leg Press (10-20 reps)															
Sled Squat															
Seated Leg Curl															
Machine Biceps Curls															
Standing BBL Biceps Curl															
Machine Triceps Pushaway															
Reverse Grip Triceps Pushdown															
Seated Calf															
Machine Donkey Calf															

135

Name: _____   **Routine: ADVANCED TOTAL #7   (6-20's)**   **Date:** _____

EXERCISE	WT	WT	WT	WT	WT	WT	WT	WT	WT	WT	WT	WT	WT	WT
ABS														
Hyperextensions														
(warm up) Bench Press														
BBL Flat Bench Press														
Dmb Incline Bench Press														
X-Over Incline Flys														
Dmb High Bench Row														
Close Grip Pulldown														
Cable Incline1-Arm Low Pull														
Smith Machine Seated Overhead Press														
BBL Upright Row														
High Bench Rear Laterals														
Sled Squat (10-20 reps)														
Hack Squat														
Leg Press														
Preacher BBL Curl														
Seated Dmb Biceps Curls														
Regular Triceps Pushdown														
Rope Triceps Pushaway														
Seated Calf														
Machine Donkey Calf														

136

EXERCISE	WT	WT	WT	WT	WT	WT	WT	WT	WT	WT	WT	WT	WT	WT	WT	WT
ABS & Hyperextensions																
Seated Row (12 reps)																
(10 reps)																
(8 reps)																
(4 reps)																
Dmb Flat Bench Press (12 reps)																
(10 reps)																
(8 reps)																
(4 reps)																
Seated Dmb Overhead Press (12 reps)																
(10 reps)																
(8 reps)																
Seated French Press (12 reps)																
(10 reps)																
(8 reps)																
Cable Preacher Curl (12 reps)																
(10 reps)																
(8 reps)																
Leg Press (12 reps)																
(10 reps)																
(8 reps)																
(4 reps)																
Machine Donkey Calf																

Name: _____   **Routine: ADVANCED TOTAL #9   Mass Builder**   **Date:** _____

EXERCISE	WT	WT	WT	WT	WT	WT	WT	WT	WT	WT	WT	WT	WT	WT	WT
ABS & Hyperextensions															
Machine Incline Bench Press (12 reps)															
(10 reps)															
(8 reps)															
(4 reps)															
Wide Grip Pulldown in Front (12 reps)															
(10 reps)															
(8 reps)															
(4 reps)															
Machine Triceps Pushaway (12 reps)															
(10 reps)															
(8 reps)															
(4 reps)															
BBL Biceps Curl (12 reps)															
(10 reps)															
(8 reps)															
(4 reps)															
Sled Squat (12 reps)															
(10 reps)															
(8 reps)															
(4 reps)															
Seated Calf (30 reps)															
(20 & 15 reps)															

CHAPTER TWENTY

HEAVY LEGS

Every woman walking into our studio wants longer more shapely legs. Of course we make no pretense on making their legs longer but we do offer suggestions on how to make the legs they were born with look more attractive. Surprisingly enough developing legs that are thinner and more muscular does tend to make them appear longer.

HEAVY LEGS PROGRAMS were developed especially for those people (men or women), that have relatively small upper bodies and massive almost piano like legs. This type of body is usually thick through the hips, knees and ankles and narrow in the shoulders. Unfortunately this body type takes a great deal more work to develop a symmetrical figure than the majority of us have to deal with. On this particular workout almost all the work goes into the legs with just a few exercises for the upper body to keep it toned while the legs are reduced in size.

The work is quite intense so particular attention must be paid to any knee, ankle or back irritation. The normal method of using the Heavy Legs Program is to exercise three times a week. However at the first sign of stress of *any* kind, alternate the *Heavy Legs* Program with one of the regular *Circuit Training* routines.

If you are alternating workouts, one time you will do Heavy Legs and the next time you will do Circuit Training. That means one week you will have two days of Heavy Legs and one day of Circuit Training. The next week you will have one day of Heavy Legs and two of Circuit Training. In this manner you will recover enough from the leg work so that you will not stress any joints.

If there is still any problem with joints or muscles, discontinue Heavy Legs and go back to Circuit Training until all discomfort is gone. I know this sounds as if it is a very difficult program. It is! However it is a marvelous program for those who have the determination <u>and</u> genetic structure to do it. Results from this type of exercise plan have been quite outstanding over the years. It's just not for everyone.

Workouts should be fun. If they are not, you are doing something wrong. It is the purpose of this Manual to keep you from making mistakes that will impede your training progress.

139

Routine: CIRCUIT (To Alternate With Legs)   Date: _____

EXERCISE	WT	WT	WT	WT	WT	WT	WT	WT	WT	WT	WT	WT	WT	WT	WT	WT
ABS & Hyperextensions																
Machine Biceps Curls																
Flat Dmb Bench Press																
Seated Leg Curl																
Hack Squat																
Incline Dmb Flys																
Seated Row (high grip)																
X-over Lying Rear Laterals																
Machine Incline Bench Press																
Seated Calf																
Wide Grip Pulldown in Front																
Leg Extension																
Pec Deck																
I Arm Dmb Row																
Seated BBL Overhead Press																
Lying Dmb French Press																
Seated Dmb Biceps Curls																
Leaning 1-arm Side Laterals																
Rope Pushdown																
Cable Lying Biceps Curls																
Machine Shoulder Shrugs																
Donkey Calf																
Dmb Kickbacks																

Name: _____

Routine: HEAVY LEGS #1 (Alternate w/Circuit)   Date: _____

EXERCISE	WT	WT	WT	WT	WT	WT	WT	WT	WT	WT	WT	WT	WT
ABS & Hyperextensions													
Dmb Swing													
Step up Lunges													
Seated Calf													
Flat Lunges													
Incline Dmb Bench Press													
Side Leg Machine in/out													
Leg Press (low plate)													
Leg Press Calves (toes out)													
Wide Grip Pulldown in Front													
Sled Squat (feet straight)													
Machine Donkey Calf													
BBL Upright Row													
Sissy Squat													
Regular Triceps Pushdown													
Side Leg Machine to Back													
Leg Press (high plate wide)													
Leg Press Calf (toes in)													
Seated French Press													
Sled Squat (toes out)													
BBL Biceps Curl													
Regular Squats-wide stance													

141

EXERCISE	WT	WT	WT	WT	WT	WT	WT	WT	WT	WT	WT	WT	WT	WT	WT	WT
ABS & Hyperextensions																
Side Leg Machine in/out																
Side Leg Machine to Back																
Lunge																
Incline Dmb Flys																
Seated Row																
Seated Calf																
Leg Extension																
Seated Leg Curl																
Hack Squat																
Machine Donkey Calf																
Incline Machine Press (10 then 20 repetitions)																
Seated Dmb Biceps Curls																
Lying BBL French Curl																
Lying Leg Curl																
Sissy Squat																
Sled Squat (10 then 30 repetitions)																
Seated Arnold Dmb Overhead Press																
Rope Pushdown (descend)																
Leg Press																
(Descending Set)																
Bent Arm Pullover																

Name: _____   Routine: **HEAVY LEGS #3**   Date: _____

EXERCISE	WT	WT	WT	WT	WT	WT	WT	WT	WT	WT	WT	WT	WT	WT	WT	WT	WT
ABS & HYPEREXTENSIONS																	
Dmb Swing																	
Lunge																	
Straight Arm Pullover																	
Leg Extensions																	
Seated BBL Overhead Press																	
Wide Pulldown in Front																	
Lying Leg Curl																	
Leg Machine in & out																	
Leg Press																	
Leg Press Calf																	
Flat BBL Bench Press																	
Machine Biceps Curls																	
Seated Leg Curl																	
Lying Dmb French Press																	
Pec Deck																	
Seated Dmb Biceps Curls																	
Sled Squat																	
Seated Calf																	
Rope Pushdown																	
Dmb Side Lateral Raises																	
Hack Squat																	

EXERCISE	WT	WT	WT	WT	WT	WT	WT	WT	WT	WT	WT	WT	WT	WT
ABS														
Hyperextensions														
BBL Clean & Press														
Leg Extensions														
Seated Leg Curl														
Incline Dmb Bench Press														
Close Grip Pulldown														
Leg Press (low plate)														
Leg Press Calf														
Hack Squat (feet close)														
Machine Donkey Calf														
Pec Deck														
Lunge														
Seated Calf														
Preacher BBL Biceps Curls														
Regular Triceps Pushdown														
Side Leg Machine in/out														
Dmb Concentration Curls														
Dmb 1-arm Kickback														
Sled Squat (legs wide)														
Leg Press (high plate)														
Side Leg Machine to Back														

CHAPTER TWENTY-ONE

SPLIT TRAINING

There comes a time in your training that working out the whole body three times a week just isn't getting the results you want. You seem to have reached a plateau in your training. You're not gaining muscle, the weights are not increasing, and you're not looking forward to your workouts. It's time to try SPLIT ROUTINES.

If the workouts are spread over four days rather than three, more sets can be done for each body part. For example, if you work the chest, deltoids, biceps and thighs one day; and the back, triceps and calves the next, *splitting your routine in half*, you can increase the number of sets you are doing for those muscles and still have more recovery time between body parts.

Changing your program in this manner should make you see rapid improvement. The first thing you will notice on this new program is that your muscles will feel more *pumped*. Doing more sets per body part will make the blood rush into the area and make the muscles feel gorged. Most people like the feeling, and the muscles will look larger. The pumped state will only last for a little while but with regular training the increased size will become permanent.

It is not a good idea to stay on a split routine for long periods of time. When you reach a plateau this time, go back to three days a week for a while. When I suggest this to people at our studio, they always complain they will not get the results they're after if they drop back to three days.

This is not true! The body must have time to recover. The only time I encourage a person to train five or six days a week is if they are getting ready for a contest or a photography session. When they are on this hard a program, they are no longer interested in gaining size or strength. Definition is the only goal you are after when you work with that much *intensity* with little recovery time allowed.

The key word here is *intensity*. When the workout is sluggish or so easy you don't even have to grab a quick breath to keep going, you can spend six days a week in the gym three hours a day and never show signs of stress. If you have ever visited a gym with any regularity, you have seen many people like this. They come to the gym year after year and never look any different than the day of their first workout. The body builders that work out with *intensity*, seldom work out more than an hour or, at the most, an hour and a half, and they are the ones that seem to grow with each passing month!

Another advantage of going back and forth between the three-day and four-day routines is the body never has a chance to adapt to the training routines. Remember the more you can confuse the muscles the more they will continue to respond. The famous magazine tycoon, Joe Weider, calls this his *"Muscle Confusion"* technique. I don't know whether he really thought of it first, I just know it works.

Name: _____   **Routine: SUPER SETS #1 - Back**   **Date:** _____

EXERCISE	WT	WT	WT	WT	WT	WT	WT	WT	WT	WT	WT	WT	WT	WT	WT
ABS															
Hyperextensions															
⎡ BBL Bent Over Row															
⎣ Cable 1-arm High Pulldown															
⎡ Bent Arm Pullover															
⎣ Cable Incline 1-arm Pull Up															
⎡ Straight Arm Pushdown															
⎣ One Arm Dmb Rows															
⎡ Straight Arm Pullover															
⎣ Dead Lift															
⎡ Alternate Dmb French Press															
⎣ Dip Between Benches															
⎡ Dmb Lying French Press															
⎣ BBL Close Grip Bench Press															
⎡ Triceps Rope Pushdown															
⎣ Cable 1-arm Pushdown															
⎡ Leg Extension															
⎣ Leg Press															
⎡ Lying Leg Curl															
⎣ Hack Squat															
⎡ Seated Leg Curl															
⎣ Sled Squat															

Name: _____   **Routine: SUPER SETS #1 Chest**   **Date:** _____

EXERCISE	WT	WT	WT	WT	WT	WT	WT	WT	WT	WT	WT	WT	WT	WT	WT	WT
Abs & Hyperextensions																
Warm Up Chest																
Machine Incline Bench Press																
Dmb Flat Bench Press																
BBL Flat Bench Press																
Dmb Incline Bench Press																
Parrillo Dips																
Push Ups																
X-over Incline Rear Laterals																
Dmb Seated Overhead Press																
X-over Lying Rear Laterals																
Dmb Side Lateral Raises																
X-over Bent Over Laterals																
Dmb Front Laterals																
Machine Biceps Curls																
Dmb Seated Biceps Curls																
Cable Preacher Biceps Curls																
BBL Preacher Curls																
Seated Calf																
Leg Press Calf																
Machine Donkey Calves																
Leg Press Calves																

147

Name: _____   Routine: SUPER SETS #2 - Back   Date: _____

EXERCISE	WT	WT	WT	WT	WT	WT	WT	WT	WT	WT	WT	WT	WT	WT	WT	WT
ABS & Hyperextensions																
Warm Up Pulldowns																
Round Grip Pulldown																
Seated Row Machine																
Close Grip Pulldown																
High Bench Dmb Row																
Reverse Grip Pulldown																
BBL High Bench Row																
Either Wide Grip Pulldown or Close Grip Pull-Up																
High Bench Reverse Grip BBL Row																
Machine Triceps Pushaway																
Regular Triceps Pushdown																
Lying BBL Triceps Kickback																
Reverse Grip Triceps Pushdown																
Rope Triceps Pushaway																
Cable Incline Kickback																
Leg Extensions																
Seated Leg Curl																
Leg Press																
Hack Squat																
Leg Press																
Sled Squat																

148

Name: _____   Routine: _____   SUPER SETS #2 - Chest   Date: _____

EXERCISE	WT	WT	WT	WT	WT	WT	WT	WT	WT	WT	WT	WT	WT	WT	WT	WT
ABS & Hyperextensions																
(warm up) Chest																
Dmb Round the World																
Dmb Fly & Press Combo																
BBL Flat Bench Press																
Dmb Incline Bench Press																
X-over Standing Fly																
Cable 1-arm Fly																
X-over Lying Rear Laterals																
Incline BBL Front Laterals																
X-over Incline Rear Laterals																
Dmb Side Lateral Raises																
Incline Dmb Front Laterals																
High Bench Rear Laterals																
High Bench Dmb Curls																
Hanging Incline BBL Curls																
Cable Preacher Curls																
Cable Lying Biceps Curls																
Seated Calf																
Leg Press Calf																
Machine Donkey Calf																
Leg Press Calf																

149

EXERCISE	WT	WT	WT	WT	WT	WT	WT	WT	WT	WT	WT	WT	WT	WT	WT	WT
Abs																
Warm Up Back																
Wide Pulldown in Front																
Seated Row																
Wide Pulldown in Front																
Dmb Bent Arm Pullover																
Wide Pulldown in Front																
Close Grip Pulldown																
Wide Pulldown in Front																
High Bench Dmb Rows																
Seated Dmb Overhead Press																
X-Over Lying Rear Laterals																
Seated Dmb Overhead Press																
X-Over Bent Over Laterals																
Seated Dmb Overhead Press																
Dmb Side Lateral Raises																
Machine Donkey Calf																
Seated Calf																
Regular Triceps Pushdown																
Seated Dmb French Press																
Regular Triceps Pushdown																
Machine Triceps Pushaway																
Regular Triceps Pushdown																
Cable Incline Kickbacks																

Name: _____   Routine: **SUPER SETS #3   Chest**   Date: _____

EXERCISE	WT	WT	WT	WT	WT	WT	WT	WT	WT	WT	WT	WT	WT	WT	WT	WT
ABS #1, 2, 3 (Alternate)																
Hyperextensions																
warm up X-over Flys																
⬒ X-Over Incline Flys																
Machine Incline Press																
⬒ X-Over Incline Flys																
Dmb Flat Bench Press																
⬒ X-Over Incline Flys																
Dmb Incline Bench Press																
⬒ Parrillo Dips																
Push-Ups																
⬒ Leg Extension																
Hack Squat																
⬒ Leg Extension																
Sled Squat																
⬒ Seated Leg Curl																
Leg Press																
⬒ Machine Biceps Curls																
Seated Dmb Biceps Curls																
⬒ Machine Biceps Curls																
Cable Preacher Biceps Curls																
⬒ Machine Biceps Curls																
Standing BBL Biceps Curls																

151

EXERCISE	WT	WT	WT	WT	WT	WT	WT	WT	WT	WT	WT	WT	WT	WT	WT	WT
ABS & Hyperextensions																
(warm up) Seated Dmb Press																
(warm up) Dmb Hanging Cleans																
Seated Dmb Overhead Press																
Dmb Hanging Cleans																
X-over Lying Rear Laterals																
Dmb Shoulder Shrugs																
X-over Incline Rear Laterals																
Dmb Side Lateral Raises																
Seated Dmb Biceps Curls																
Regular Triceps Pushdown																
Machine Biceps Curls																
Machine Triceps Pushaway																
Cable Preacher Biceps Curls																
Seated Dmb French Press																
Standing BBL Biceps Curls																
X-over Incline Kickbacks																
Seated Calf																
Machine Donkey Calf																
Leg Press Calf																
Seated Calf																
Machine Donkey Calf																
Leg Press Calf																

EXERCISE	WT	WT	WT	WT	WT	WT	WT	WT	WT	WT	WT	WT	WT	WT	WT	WT
ABS																
Hyperextensions																
(warm up) Machine Incline Press																
(warm up) Wide Grip Pulldown chin																
(Do All upper super-sets once before repeating 2X)																
Machine Incline Press																
Wide Grip Pulldown to Chin																
Dmb Flat Bench Press																
Seated Row																
X-over Incline Flys																
Close Grip Pulldown																
(Do All lower super-sets then repeat the 2 marked)																
Leg Extension																
SeatedLeg Curl																
Leg Press																
Hack Squat																
Lying Leg Curl																
Sled Squat																

153

Name: _____   Routine: **SUPER SETS #5 Push-Pull (part 1)**   Date: _____

EXERCISE	WT	WT	WT	WT	WT	WT	WT	WT	WT	WT	WT	WT	WT	WT	WT	WT
ABS																
Dmb Clean & Press																
Incline BBL Press																
Round Grip Pulldown																
Decline BBL Bench Press																
Close Grip Pulldown																
Flat BBL Bench Press																
High Bench Dmb Row																
Push Ups																
Pull Ups																
Peck Deck																
Dead Lift																
Hyperextensions																
Good Mornings																
Dmb Front Lateral Raise																
Incline Dmb Rear Laterals																
Incline BBL Front Laterals																
Side Lateral Raises																
X-Over Lying Rear Laterals																
Seated Dmb Overhead Press																

Name: _____ **Routine: SUPER SETS #5 Push-Pull (part 2) Date:** _____

EXERCISE	WT	WT	WT	WT	WT	WT	WT	WT	WT	WT	WT	WT	WT	WT	WT	WT
ABS																
Hyperextensions																
Leg Press (warm up)																
⌐Leg Extension																
└Leg Curl																
Sissy Squat																
⌐Leg Press																
└Sled Squat																
Lunge																
⌐Hack Squat																
└Leg Press																
Sled Squat																
Standing Alternate ⌐Dmb Biceps Curl																
└Triceps Pushdown																
Wall BBL Biceps Curls																
⌐Machine Triceps Pushaway																
└Seated Dmb Hammer Curls																
Rope Triceps Pushdown																
⌐Seated Calf																
└Leg Press Calf																
Machine Donkey Calf																

155

Name: _____   Routine: Descending #1 Split Back   Date: _____

EXERCISE	WT	WT	WT	WT	WT	WT	WT	WT	WT	WT	WT	WT	WT	WT	WT	WT
ABS & Hyperextensions																
Warm Up Back																
Wide Pulldown in Front																
Descending Set																
High Dmb Bench Row																
Descending Set																
Cable 1-arm Hi Pulldown																
Descending Set																
Leg Extension																
Seated Leg Curl																
Sled Squat																
Descending Set																
Leg Press																
Descending Set																
Reverse Grip Pushdown																
Descending Set																
BBL Lying French Press																
Descending Set																
Cable Incline Kickbacks																
Descending Set																
Leg Press Calf																
Machine Donkey Calf																

EXERCISE	WT	WT	WT	WT	WT	WT	WT	WT	WT	WT	WT	WT	WT	WT	WT	WT
ABS & Hyperextensions																
Warm Up Chest																
Machine Incline Bench Press																
Descending Set																
Smith Flat Bench Press																
Descending Set																
Flat Dmb Flys																
Descending Set																
Parrillo Dips																
Machine Overhead Press																
Descending Set																
X-over Lying Rear Laterals																
Descending Set																
Cable Upright Rows																
Descending Set																
Cable Lying Biceps Curls																
Descending Set																
Hanging Incline Dmb Curls																
Descending Set																
Preacher BBL Biceps Curls																
Descending Set																
Machine Donkey Calf																
Seated Calf																

Routine: Descending #2 Split Back

EXERCISE	WT	WT	WT	WT	WT	WT	WT	WT	WT	WT	WT	WT	WT	WT	WT
ABS & Hyperextensions															
Warm Up Back															
Round Grip Pulldown															
Close Grip Pull Ups															
Cable 1-arm High Pulldown															
Cable Incline Low 1-arm Pull															
Round Grip Pulldown															
Descending Set															
Seated Row															
Descending Set															
Machine Donkey Calf															
Leg Press Calf															
X-over Incline Rear Laterals															
Descending Set															
Dmb Side Lateral Raises															
Descending Set															
Machine Overhead Press															
Descending Sets															
Rope Triceps Pushdown															
Descending Set															
Rope Overhead Pushaway															
Descending Set															

EXERCISE	WT	WT	WT	WT	WT	WT	WT	WT	WT	WT	WT	WT	WT	WT
ABS														
Hyperextensions														
Warm Up Chest														
Incline Dmb Bench Press														
Flat Dmb Bench Press														
Machine Incline Bench Press														
Descending Set														
X-over Incline Flys														
Descending Set														
Seated Dmb Curls														
BBL Biceps Curls														
Machine Biceps Curls														
Descending Set														
Preacher BBL Curls														
Descending Set														
Leg Extension														
Seated Leg Curl														
Sled Squat														
Descending Set														
Leg Press														
Descending Set														

159

EXERCISE	WT	WT	WT	WT	WT	WT	WT	WT	WT	WT	WT	WT	WT	WT
ABS & Hyperextensions														
Warm Up Back														
Close Grip Pull Ups														
Close Grip Pulldown														
Wide Grip Pull Up														
Wide Grip Pulldown														
Seated Row														
descending set														
Wide Grip Upright Row														
descending set														
Seated Dmb Overhead Press														
descending set														
Side Lateral Raises														
descending sets														
Cable Seated French Press														
descending set														
Machine Triceps Pushaway														
descending set														
Regular Triceps Pushdown														
descending set														
Machine Shrugs														
descending set														

EXERCISE	WT	WT	WT	WT	WT	WT	WT	WT	WT	WT	WT	WT	WT	WT	WT	WT	WT
Abs & Hyperextensions																	
Warm Up Chest																	
Dmb Incline Flys																	
descending set																	
Dmb Incline Press																	
descending set																	
Pec Deck																	
descending set																	
Leg Extensions																	
Leg Press																	
descending set																	
Hack Squat																	
descending set																	
Sled Squat																	
descending set																	
Cable Preacher Biceps Curls																	
descending set																	
BBL Biceps Curls																	
descending set																	
Concentration Biceps Curls																	
descending set																	

Routine: Ascending #1 Split   Back 30 second rest   **Date: _____**

#	EXERCISE	WT	WT	WT	WT	WT	WT	WT	WT	WT	WT	WT	WT	WT	WT	WT	WT
	ABS & Hyperextensions																
11	Seated Row																
	Ascending set																
10	Pulldown Round Grip																
	Ascending set																
32	Incline 1-Arm Cable Pull Up																
	Ascending set																
18	Triceps Pushdown																
	Ascending set																
16	Machine Pushaway																
	Ascending set																
32	Cable Incline Kickbacks																
	ascending set																
22	Leg Extensions twice																
23	Seated Leg Curl twice																
	Leg Press																
	Ascending set																
25	Hack Squat																
	Ascending set																
27	Seated Calf																
	Ascending set																
21	Leg Press Calf - Ascending																

162

Name: _____   Routine: Ascending #1 Split Chest 30 second rest   Date: _____

# EXERCISE	WT	WT	WT	WT	WT	WT	WT	WT	WT	WT	WT	WT	WT	WT
ABS & Hyperextensions														
X-over Flat Flys														
Ascending set														
1 Machine Incline Bench Press														
Ascending set														
2 Dmb Incline Bench Press														
Ascending set														
32 X-over Lying Rear Laterals														
Ascending set														
BBL Upright Row														
Ascending set														
32 X-over Incline Rear Laterals														
14 Machine Biceps Curls														
Ascending set														
2 Dmb Incline Bench Curls														
Ascending set														
32 Cable Lying Biceps Curls														
Ascending set														
22 Leg Extension														
Ascending set														
29 Machine Donkey Calf														
21 Leg Press & Calf														

163

Routine: 6-20's #1   SPLIT - Back

EXERCISE	WT	WT	WT	WT	WT	WT	WT	WT	WT	WT	WT	WT	WT	WT	WT
ABS															
Hyperextensions															
Warm Up Back															
Wide Pulldown to Chin 6-20															
Seated Row 6-20															
Close Grip Pulldown 6-20															
Dmb High Bench Row 6-20															
Warm Up Legs															
Leg Extension															
Seated Leg Curl															
Hack Squat															
(10 - 15 - 20 Repetitions)															
Reverse Grip Pushdown 6-20															
Lying BBL French Press 6-20															
Rope Overhead Pushaway															
Incline Cable Kickbacks															
Triceps Bench Dips															
Seated Calf															
Machine Donkey Calf															
Dmb Biceps Curls															
BBL Biceps Curls															
Regular Pull Ups															

Name: _____   **Routine: 6 - 20's #1   Split - Chest**   **Date:** _____

EXERCISE	WT	WT	WT	WT	WT	WT	WT	WT	WT	WT	WT	WT	WT	WT	WT
ABS & Hyperextensions															
Warm Up Flat Flys															
Flat Dmb Bench Flys 6-20															
Machine Incline Press 6-20															
Flat BBL Bench Press 6-20															
Incline Dmb Press 6-20															
Parallel Dips															
Warm Up Legs															
Leg Press 6-20															
Sled Squat 6-20															
Hack Squat 6-20															
Seated Dmb Press 6-20															
Leaning Side Laterals 6-20															
Machine Shrugs 6-20															
BBL Preacher Curls 6-20															
BBL Biceps Curls 6-20															
High Bench Dmb Biceps Curls 6-20															
Cable Concentration Curls 6-20															

Name: _____ **Routine:** **GIANT SETS - SPLIT #1 Back (3 in a row) Date:** _____

EXERCISE	WT	WT	WT	WT	WT	WT	WT	WT	WT	WT	WT	WT	WT	WT	WT
ABS															
Hyperextensions															
(Warm Up Back)															
Wide Pulldown in Front															
Seated Row															
Cable 1-arm High Pulldown															
Round Grip Pulldown															
BBL Bent Over Row															
Cable Incline Low 1-arm Pull															
Regular Triceps Pushdown															
Seated Dmb French Press															
Machine Triceps Pushaway															
Reverse Grip Pushdown															
Rope Overhead Pushaway															
Cable Incline Kickbacks															
Sled Squat															
Hack Squat															
Leg Press															
Seated Leg Curl															
Leg Extension															
Leg Press															

166

EXERCISE	WT	WT	WT	WT	WT	WT	WT	WT	WT	WT	WT	WT	WT	WT	WT
ABS															
Hyperextensions															
(Warm Up Chest)															
Machine Incline Bench Press															
Flat Dmb Bench Press															
Incline Dmb Bench Press															
Flat BBL Bench Press															
Parrillo Dips															
Push Ups															
X-over Bent Over Laterals															
Dmb Side Laterals															
X-over Incline Rear Laterals															
X-over Lying Rear Laterals															
Dmb Side Laterals															
Dmb Front Laterals															
Machine Biceps Curls															
Cable Preacher Biceps Curls															
Seated Dmb Biceps Curls															
Cable Lying Biceps Curls															
BBL Preacher Biceps Curls															
BBL Reverse Grip Curls															
Machine Donkey Calf															
Seated Calf															
Leg Press Calf															

167

EXERCISE	WT	WT	WT	WT	WT	WT	WT	WT	WT	WT	WT	WT	WT	WT
Abs & Hyperextensions														
Wide Pulldown in Front														
Seated Row														
Bent Arm Pullover														
Close Grip Pulldown														
Straight Arm Pullover														
High Dmb Bench Row														
Regular Triceps Pushdown														
Machine Pushaway														
Seated French Press														
Lying BBL Kickbacks														
Rope Pushaway														
Cable Incline Kickbacks														
Machine Biceps Curls														
Cable Preacher Curls														
Standing Dmb Curls														
Reverse Grip BBL Curls														
Standing BBL Curls														
Hanging Incline BBL Curls														

Name: _____ **Routine: Giant Sets #2 Split   Chest   (6 In a Row)**   **Date:** _____

EXERCISE	WT	WT	WT	WT	WT	WT	WT	WT	WT	WT	WT	WT	WT	WT	WT	WT
Abs & Hyperextensions																
X-over Incline Flys																
Flat Dmb Bench Press																
Machine Incline Bench Press																
Flat BBL Bench Press																
Incline Dmb Bench Press																
Incline Dmb Flys																
X-over Lying Rear Laterals																
Side Lateral Raises																
Seated Dmb Overhead Press																
High Bench Rear Laterals																
X-over Bent Over Laterals																
Machine Shrugs																
Leg Extension																
Leg Curl																
Hack Squat																
Leg Press																
Sled Squat																
Sissy Squat																
Leg Press Calf																
Seated Calf																

169

#	EXERCISE	WT	WT	WT	WT	WT	WT	WT	WT	WT	WT	WT	WT	WT	WT	WT	WT	WT
	ABS & Hyperextensions																	
	(warm up) Wide Pulldown Shrugs																	
	(warm up) Seated Row Shrugs																	
	Wide Pulldown Shrugs																	
	Seated Row																	
	Close Grip Pulldown																	
	High Bench Dmb Row																	
	Bent Arm Pullover																	
	Dmb Shoulder Shrugs																	
	Machine Shrugs																	
	Dmb Shrugs																	
	Regular Triceps Pushdown																	
	Machine Triceps Pushaway																	
	Seated Dmb French Press																	
	Cable Incline Kickbacks																	
	Sled Squat																	
	Leg Press																	
	Seated Leg Curl																	
	Machine Donkey Calf																	
	Seated Calf																	
	Leg Press Calf																	
	Minutes to Complete W/O																	

170

Name: _____ **Routine:** _____ **TIMED WORKOUT #1 Split Chest** **Date:** _____

EXERCISE	WT	WT	WT	WT	WT	WT	WT	WT	WT	WT	WT	WT	WT	WT	WT	WT
ABS & Hyperextensions																
(warm up) Incline Flys																
(warm up) Incline Press																
X-over Incline Flys																
Machine Incline Bench Press																
(palms in) Dmb Flat Bench Press																
(palms in) Dmb Incline Bench Press																
BBL Flat Bench Press																
Parrillo Dips																
X-over Lying Rear Laterals																
Dmb Side Laterals																
Seated Dmb Overhead Press																
X-over Incline Rear Laterals																
Machine Biceps Curls																
Cable Preacher Biceps Curl																
BBL Biceps Curl																
Reverse Grip BBL Curl																
Leg Extension																
Seated Leg Curl																
Sled Squat																
Hack Squat																
Leg Press																
Minutes to Complete W/O																

Be Careful Not To Overtrain

Signs of Overtraining Are:

Irritability

Difficulty Sleeping

Loss of Appetite

172

CHAPTER TWENTY-TWO

HEAVY TRAINING

When you are ready for a challenging workout, **HEAVY TRAINING** is for you! The idea for these workouts came from an article that appeared in "Muscle and Fitness Magazine" written by Larry Scott, the first Mr. Olympia. He claims it's the best workout he ever came up with and I have to agree. It is my favorite program as well.

HEAVY TRAINING is done as a split routine. The main difference between this and some of the other similar programs in this manual is that when you go to the set that is for one or two repetitions only, you must use a weight that scares you! A training partner is an absolute requirement when trying this workout.

On these heavy training routines always take as much time as you need to warm up. Take a weight that you can easily handle for twelve repetitions for your first warm up set. Then try another set after a short rest, but this time use a heavier poundage that you can easily do for eight reps. It is not necessary to record your warm up weights. Most of us here at **FOREVER YOUNG** do at least two sets to get the muscles going. If it is unusually cold or you are feeling sluggish, do as many as you need before trying the heavier weights.

The first set of twenty repetitions requires a weight that normally uses ninety percent of your maximum capabilities. If you reach your goal of twenty reps the next workout, you must increase the resistance. For example, if you are doing the flat bench press with one hundred pounds and you knock out twenty repetitions, the next workout you must go to at least one hundred and two and a half pounds. That procedure is true of all the sets you do on this Heavy Duty program.

The next set of six to eight repetitions goes to failure. Pick a weight that you think you can do six times and shoot for eight repetitions. If you hit eight repetitions, you must increase the poundages the next day you try this movement. On this program every time you hit your mark *in good form*, the weights have to go up.

The big set, the set that scares you, is where your partner comes in. He has to help you complete the movement. This is the exercise that forces the muscles to grow! If you try the exercise and you are able to complete the movement unassisted for two repetitions, the weight was too light. This set is not only a test of strength, but one of courage as well!

The remaining two sets are to failure as well. If the first set of twenty repetitions was easy for you, on the final set of twenty increase the poundage. Properly done, this last exercise should be the most difficult to perform. By this time the body should be screaming for mercy. If it isn't, you're not pushing hard enough!

This program should not be attempted until you have at least six months of training under your belt. Without a training partner, you can't handle the weights necessary to get the results this kind of work demands. Keep the form strict, get scared on that high set, use a good training partner and you will be amazed by how fast your body responds.

Routine: HEAVY TRAINING #1a - Split Back   Date: _____

EXERCISE	WT	WT	WT	WT	WT	WT	WT	WT	WT	WT	WT	WT	WT	WT	WT	WT	WT	WT
ABS & Hyperextension																		
Round Grip Pulldown (20 reps)																		
(8 reps)																		
(4 reps)																		
(12 reps)																		
(20 reps)																		
Dmb Shrugs (20 reps)																		
(8 reps)																		
(4 reps)																		
(12 reps)																		
(20 reps)																		
Regular Triceps Pushdown (20 reps)																		
(8 reps)																		
(4 reps)																		
(12 reps)																		
(20 reps)																		
Leg Press (20 reps)																		
(8 reps)																		
(4 reps)																		
(12 reps)																		
(20 reps)																		
Leg Press Calf																		

Name: _____   **Routine: HEAVY TRAINING #1a   Split Chest   Date:** _____

EXERCISE	WT	WT	WT	WT	WT	WT	WT	WT	WT	WT	WT	WT	WT	WT	WT	WT
ABS & Hyperextensions																
Flat BBL Bench Press (20 reps)																
(8 reps)																
(4 reps)																
(12 reps)																
(20 reps)																
Machine Seated Overhead Press (20 reps)																
(8 reps)																
(4 reps)																
(12 reps)																
(20 reps)																
Machine Biceps Curl (20 reps)																
(8 reps)																
(4 reps)																
(12 reps)																
(20 reps)																
Sled Squat (20 reps)																
(8 reps)																
(4 reps)																
(12 reps)																
(20 reps)																
Seated Calves																

175

Name: _____ Routine: HEAVY TRAINING #1b - Split Back Date: _____

EXERCISE	WT	WT	WT	WT	WT	WT	WT	WT	WT	WT	WT	WT	WT	WT	WT
ABS & Hyperextensions															
High Bench Dmb Row (20 reps)															
(8 reps)															
(4 reps)															
(12 reps)															
(20 reps)															
Machine Shrugs (20 reps)															
(8 reps)															
(4 reps)															
(12 reps)															
(20 reps)															
Machine Triceps Pushaway (20 reps)															
(8 reps)															
(4 reps)															
(12 reps)															
(20 reps)															
Seated Leg Curl (20 reps)															
(8 reps)															
(4 reps)															
(12 reps)															
(20 reps)															
Machine Donkey Calf															

EXERCISE	WT	WT	WT	WT	WT	WT	WT	WT	WT	WT	WT	WT	WT	WT	WT	WT	WT	WT
ABS & Hyperextensions																		
Machine Incline Bench Press (20 reps)																		
(8 reps)																		
(4 reps)																		
(12 reps)																		
(20 reps)																		
Seated Dmb Overhead Press (20 reps)																		
(8 reps)																		
(4 reps)																		
(12 reps)																		
(20 reps)																		
Cable Preacher Biceps Curls (20 reps)																		
(8 reps)																		
(4 reps)																		
(12 reps)																		
(20 reps)																		
Hack Squat (20 reps)																		
(8 reps)																		
(4 reps)																		
(12 reps)																		
(20 reps)																		

Name: _____   **Routine: HEAVY TRAINING #2a - Split Back**   **Date:** _____

EXERCISE	WT	WT	WT	WT	WT	WT	WT	WT	WT	WT	WT	WT	WT	WT	WT	WT
ABS & Hyperextensions																
Pulldown in Front (20 reps)																
(6-8 reps)																
(1-2 reps)																
(10-12 reps)																
(20 reps)																
Regular Triceps Pushdown (20 reps)																
(6-8 reps)																
(1-2 reps)																
(10-12 reps)																
(20 reps)																
Leg Press - High Plate (20 reps)																
(6-8 reps)																
(1-2 reps)																
(10-12 reps)																
(20 reps)																
Machine Shrugs (20 reps)																
(6-8 reps)																
(1-2 reps)																
(10-12 reps)																
(20 reps)																

Name: _____   **Routine: HEAVY TRAINING #2a - Split Chest   Date:** _____

EXERCISE	WT	WT	WT	WT	WT	WT	WT	WT	WT	WT	WT	WT	WT	WT	WT	WT
ABS																
Good Mornings																
Machine Incline Bench Press (20 reps)																
(6-8 reps)																
(1-2 reps)																
(10-12 reps)																
(20 reps)																
Seated Machine Overhead Press (20 reps)																
(6-8 reps)																
(1-2 reps)																
(10-12 reps)																
(20 reps)																
Machine Biceps Curls (20 reps)																
(6-8 reps)																
(1-2 reps)																
(10-12 reps)																
(20 reps)																
Machine Donkey Calf (20 reps)																
(6-8 reps)																
(1-2 reps)																
(10-12 reps)																
(20 reps)																

EXERCISE	WT	WT	WT	WT	WT	WT	WT	WT	WT	WT	WT	WT	WT	WT	WT	WT	WT
ABS & Hyperextensions																	
Seated Row (20 reps)																	
(6-8 reps)																	
(1-2 reps)																	
(10-12 reps)																	
(20 reps)																	
Machine Triceps Pushaway (20 reps)																	
(6-8 reps)																	
(1-2 reps)																	
(10-12 reps)																	
(20 reps)																	
Sled Squat (20 reps)																	
(6-8 reps)																	
(1-2 reps)																	
(10-12 reps)																	
(20 reps)																	
Hanging BBL Clean (20 reps)																	
(6-8 reps)																	
(1-2 reps)																	
(10-12 reps)																	
(20 reps)																	

Routine: HEAVY TRAINING #2b - Split Chest   Date: _____

EXERCISE	WT	WT	WT	WT	WT	WT	WT	WT	WT	WT	WT	WT	WT	WT	WT
ABS															
Good Mornings															
X-over Incline Flys (20 reps)															
(6-8 reps)															
(1-2 reps)															
10-12 reps)															
(20 reps)															
X-over Lying Rear Laterals (20 reps)															
(6-8 reps)															
(1-2 reps)															
10-12 reps)															
(20 reps)															
BBL Biceps Curl (20 reps)															
(6-8 reps)															
(1-2 reps)															
10-12 reps)															
(20 reps)															
Leg Press Calf (30 reps)															
(20 reps)															
(6-8 reps)															
(20 reps)															

EXERCISE	WT	WT	WT	WT	WT	WT	WT	WT	WT	WT	WT	WT	WT	WT	WT	WT
ABS																
Hyperextensions																
Close Grip Pulldown (20 reps)																
(6-8 reps)																
(1-2 reps)																
(10-12 reps)																
(20 reps)																
Lying BBL French Press (20 reps)																
(6-8 reps)																
(1-2 reps)																
(10-12 reps)																
(20 reps)																
Hack Squat (20 reps)																
(6-8 reps)																
(1-2 reps)																
(10-12 reps)																
(20 reps)																
Dmb Shrugs (20 reps)																
(6-8 reps)																
(1-2 reps)																
(10-12 reps)																
(20 reps)																

EXERCISE	WT	WT	WT	WT	WT	WT	WT	WT	WT	WT	WT	WT	WT	WT	WT	WT	WT
ABS																	
Good Mornings																	
Flat Dmb Bench Press (20 reps)																	
(6-8 reps)																	
(1-2 reps)																	
(10-12 reps)																	
(20 reps)																	
Seated Dmb Overhead Press (20 reps)																	
(6-8 reps)																	
(1-2 reps)																	
(10-12 reps)																	
(20 reps)																	
Cable Preacher Biceps Curls (20 reps)																	
(6-8 reps)																	
(1-2 reps)																	
(10-12 reps)																	
(20 reps)																	
Seated Calf (20 reps)																	
(6-8 reps)																	
(1-2 reps)																	
(10-12 reps)																	
(20 reps)																	

CHAPTER TWENTY-THREE

HOME TRAINING

Judging from all the businesses selling home gym equipment, many people today prefer to train at home. You certainly can save lots of time by not having to drive to a gym. There are no lines waiting for equipment at home. You eliminate the bulging hulks and thong clad beauties that seem to proliferate most of the Spa type gyms. If the weight room is a family affair, workouts can be a fun activity.

The home routines listed in this manual are for home gyms with only the most basic of equipment. You can get a lot done with just a barbell, a set of dumbbells and an adjustable bench. When I started training I made a set of dumbbells with empty tin cans filled with cement and sections of a broom I cut up to use as handles for my dumbbells. A wooden orange crate was my bench, and I used bricks on one end to make the bench an adjustable incline bench. It was pretty primitive, but it worked!

I always preferred working out in a gym. The camaraderie I developed with my training partners was always gratifying to me and the competition we developed between ourselves made us work harder. But that is me. There are those who would never have done training alone at home. I enjoyed competition both as a body builder and as a power lifter so the gym was a great place for me to have fun.

contests, he went back to home training and was still able to maintain a magnificent body.

Complete home gyms are costly. If you are not quite sure which way to go, most gyms will allow you a trial period at little or no cost. Weigh the pros and cons before making a large purchase. Usually, you can train at a gym or health club for many years for what it would cost to buy a complete home gym. The health club can be like a private island away from children, phones and annoying neighbors. On the other hand the music can be blaring, sweaty bodies can be a problem and then there are those imposing hulks and the thong bikini babes!

There is also the personal training gym. These fitness centers are usually much quieter, more organized, the staff is often better trained. Since you would probably pay by the hour, the staff is anxious to please you. If you don't get the results you want, you will leave. The personal training gym costs more but the service, if you can afford it, is worth the money.

If you intend to train at home, a few sessions with private instruction could help you avoid many pitfalls and muscle soreness.

No matter where you train whether at home or at a professional gym, the results you get will be in direct ratio to the enthusiasm you bring to the training session. Set goals. Give yourself time limits to reach those goals. If possible, get a training partner. Most important, be consistent in your training and stick to the programs in the manual. Keep records of the weights and repetitions used in the workouts. Then just watch the transformation and enjoy!

Another man I knew, who was just two days younger than I, loved working out at home. In his first physique competition he easily walked away with the winner's trophy. The other contestants wondered at how he could work out alone and still win the contest so easily.The man's name was Vic Seipke, and he continued to win many physique titles. During the remainder of his competitive days he did join the Y.M.C.A. where most of the hard core body builders then trained. When he retired from the physique

Name: _____

Routine: **Home Workout #1**   w/Super-Sets   Date: _____

EXERCISE	WT	WT	WT	WT	WT	WT	WT	WT	WT	WT	WT	WT	WT	WT
ABS #1,2 & 3														
Dmb Swing														
BBL Flat Bench Press														
Dmb Incline Bench Press														
BBL Flat Bench Press														
Dmb Incline Bench Press														
One Leg Calf Raise														
Wide Grip Pulldown														
Close Grip Pulldown														
Wide Grip Pulldown														
Cable Incline 1-arm Pull Up														
Alternate Leg Lunge														
Regular Dmb Squats														
Alternate Leg Lunge														
Regular Dmb Squats														
BBL Biceps Curls														
Standing Alternate Dmb Biceps Curls														
Regular Triceps Pushdown														
Rope Overhead Pushaway														
Cable Biceps Curls														
Dmb Alternate French Press														

185

Name: _____ **Routine: Home Workout #2 Circuit Date:** _____

EXERCISE	WT	WT	WT	WT	WT	WT	WT	WT	WT	WT	WT	WT	WT	WT	WT	WT
Abs																
Good Mornings																
Dmb Swing																
Alternate Overhead Press																
BBL Bent Over Row																
Dmb Flat Bench Flys																
Dmb Alternate Biceps Curls																
BBL Flat Bench Press																
Dmb 1-Arm Row																
One Leg Calf Raises																
Dmb Upright Row																
BBL Lying French Press																
BBL Biceps Curls																
Dmb Shoulder Shrugs																
Dmb Lunge																
Dmb Bent Arm Pullover																
Side Lateral Raises																
Dmb Triceps Kickback																
Two Leg Calf Raise																
Squats																

Name: _____   Routine: Home Workout #3 Circuit   Date: _____

EXERCISE	WT	WT	WT	WT	WT	WT	WT	WT	WT	WT	WT	WT	WT	WT	WT
Ab Routine #2															
Dmb Clean & Press															
Dmb Bent Over Row															
Dmb Flat Bench Press															
BBL Lunge															
Dmb Seated Biceps Curls															
Seated Arnold Press															
Dmb Lying French Press															
BBL Shoulder Shrugs															
BBL Dead Lift															
Straight Arm Pullover															
Floor Push Ups															
Dmb Concentration Curls															
Dmb Front Lateral Raise															
BBL Squat															
Dmb Bent Arm Pullover															
Leaning Side Laterals															
Black Jack Curls															
Dmb Lying French Press															
1 Leg Calf Raise															
Bent Over Side Laterals															

EXERCISE	WT	WT	WT	WT	WT	WT	WT	WT	WT	WT	WT	WT	WT	WT
Ab Routine #3														
Dmb Clean & Press														
Dmb Bent Over Row														
Dmb Flat Bench Press														
BBL Lunge														
Seated Dmb Curl														
Seated Arnold Press														
Lying Dmb French Press														
BBL Dead Lift														
Straight Arm Pullover														
Floor Push Ups														
Dmb Concentration Curl														
Dmb Front Lateral Raise														
BBL Squat														
Bent Arm Pullover														
Leaning Side Lateral														
Black Jack Curls														
Lying Dmb French Press														
1 Leg Calf Raise														
Bent over Laterals														

Name: _____   Routine: Home Workout #5 Push Pull   Date: _____

EXERCISE	WT	WT	WT	WT	WT	WT	WT	WT	WT	WT	WT	WT	WT	WT	WT	WT
Ab Routine #3																
BBL Hi Pull Up																
Dmb Bent Arm Pullover																
BBL Bench Press																
BBL Bent Over Row																
Flat Dmb Fly																
Dmb Bent Over Row																
Flat Dmb Bench Press																
BBL Dead Lift																
BBL Squat																
Dmb Dead Lift																
Lunge																
Dmb Biceps Curls																
Standing BBL French Press																
Reverse Grip BBL Curls																
Bent Over Dmb Kickbacks																
Regular Grip BBL Curls																
Lying Dmb French Press																
Side Lateral Raise																
Dmb Shrugs																
Front Lateral Raise																
BBL Shrugs																

EXERCISE	WT	WT	WT	WT	WT	WT	WT	WT	WT	WT	WT	WT	WT	WT	WT
AB Routine #2															
BBL Hi Pull Up															
Dmb Bent Arm Pullover															
BBL Bench Press															
BBL Bent Over Row															
Dmb Flat Fly															
Dmb Bent over Row															
Dmb Flat Bench Press															
BBL Dead Lift															
BBL Squat															
Dmb Dead Lift															
Lunge															
Dmb Biceps Curls															
BBL Standing French Press															
BBL Reverse Grip Curls															
Dmb 2 Hand Kickback															
BBL Biceps Curls															
Dmb Lying French Press															
Side Lateral Raise															
Dmb Shrugs															
Front Lateral Raise															
BBL Shrugs															

Name: _____

Routine: Home Workout #7 Slow-Fast
(30 second rest between 1st & 2nd super-set)

Date: _____

EXERCISE	WT	WT	WT	WT	WT	WT	WT	WT	WT	WT	WT	WT	WT	WT
Abs (rotate #1,#2,#3)														
BBL Clean & Press														
slow Dmb Bent Over Row														
fast Dmb Bent Over Row														
slow BBL Bent Over Row														
fast BBL Bent Over Row														
slow Flat Dmb Fly														
fast Flat Dmb Fly														
slow Flat BBL Bench Press														
fast Flat BBL Bench Press														
slow Standing Dmb Curl														
fast Standing Dmb Curl														
slow BBl Curl														
fast BBL Curl														
slow Seated Dmb French Press														
fast Seated Dmb French Press														
slow 1 Leg Standing Calf Raise														
fast 1 Leg Standing Calf Raise														
slow BBL Dead Lift														
fast BBL Dead Lift														
slow BBL Squat														
fast BBL Squat														